I0147919

HORMONE HAVOC

ALSO BY AMY SHAH, MD

I'm So Effing Hungry

I'm So Effing Tired

HORMONE HAVOC

A SCIENCE-BACKED PROTOCOL

FOR PERIMENOPAUSE AND MENOPAUSE:

SLEEP BETTER. THINK BETTER. FEEL BETTER.

AMY SHAH, MD

HARVEST

An Imprint of WILLIAM MORROW

Without limiting the exclusive rights of any author, contributor or the publisher of this publication, any unauthorized use of this publication to train generative artificial intelligence (AI) technologies is expressly prohibited. HarperCollins also exercise their rights under Article 4(3) of the Digital Single Market Directive 2019/790 and expressly reserve this publication from the text and data mining exception.

This book contains advice and information relating to health care. It should be used to supplement rather than replace the advice of your doctor or another trained health professional. If you know or suspect you have a health problem, it is recommended that you seek your physician's advice before embarking on any medical program or treatment. All efforts have been made to assure the accuracy of the information contained in this book as of the date of publication. This publisher and the author disclaim liability for any medical outcomes that may occur as a result of applying the methods suggested in this book. Some names and identifying details have been changed.

HORMONE HAVOC. Copyright © 2026 by Amy Shah, M.D. All rights reserved. No part of this book may be used or reproduced in any manner whatsoever without written permission except in the case of brief quotations embodied in critical articles and reviews. For information, address HarperCollins Publishers, 195 Broadway, New York, NY 10007. In Europe, HarperCollins Publishers, Macken House, 39/40 Mayor Street Upper, Dublin 1, D01 C9W8, Ireland.

HarperCollins books may be purchased for educational, business, or sales promotional use. For information, please email the Special Markets Department at SPsales@harpercollins.com.

hc.com

FIRST EDITION

Library of Congress Cataloging-in-Publication Data has been applied for.

ISBN 978-0-06-342085-4

Printed in the United States of America

26 27 28 29 30 LBC 8 7 6 5 4

This book is dedicated to my "whys": Akshay, my husband, whose unwavering support turns my wildest ideas into reality; Jaden and Lara, who teach me that the best health (and life!) advice often comes from our children; and my readers, whose love and interest continue to humble and inspire me. This book is a love letter to all of you.

Contents

Introduction

Say Good-bye to Hormone Havoc

GETTING OLDER CAN BE A funny thing. I'm in my forties, and I feel anything but old. I've never been embarrassed about my age before; if anything, it's been a point of pride for me. And it has truly never occurred to me that I was anything but a young woman—I figured I had decades before anyone would look at me and think "old lady."

Life has a funny way of giving us hard reality checks when we least expect them.

For spring break in 2023, we traveled to Peru as a family. We wanted our kids to experience a backpacking expedition and to have a family trip without them on their phones the entire time. I'd been to Machu Picchu and hiked the Inca Trail for 5 days, which was a transformative experience for me. I wanted to share that with my kids. But I didn't expect to spend the trip contemplating my own mortality and facing some realities of ageism for the first time.

At the end of the 5-day hike, we stood in a circle with the entirely male crew we'd been camping and hiking with. We went around and each person said thank you and, for some reason, shared our age.

When it was my turn, I praised everyone for the beautiful food, their hospitality, and for teaching us about their culture. I also mentioned that I was forty-six. The entire circle of men gasped and started whispering to each other, and some of them were even laughing. I asked my husband, who's fluent in Spanish, what was going on, and he said, "They're surprised that you're forty-six. They thought you were much younger."

For most people, that would be a compliment. For me, it just exemplified the stigma that comes for women in their forties. I couldn't get the visual of them laughing and whispering to each other out of my head for the rest of the trip. I couldn't remember ever feeling so embarrassed at myself for something as simple as my age. I thought to myself: "I'm young! I have so much more to do!"

I'm not blaming the guides—in fact, I'm from an Indian background, and I'm familiar with the way South Asian cultures regard women in their forties as they transition to different roles in society. I know there is a cultural component to aging. Despite having a fantastic time with my family in one of the most beautiful places on the planet, this experience highlighted for me the negative ways society perceives women in their forties and older—it left me feeling frustrated. Now that I'm in my forties and am embarking on some of the hormone changes that come with this life stage, I didn't know how to feel.

While nothing about me had changed, I suddenly saw myself the way others might think of me when they learn how old I am. I started questioning myself and wondering if the best years of my life were in fact behind me. But because of my background, I didn't just wallow in this feeling but approached these questions the way I do most health-related problems. As a double-board-certified medical doctor, I wanted to see what the research had to say. I knew I was getting older and progressing along what I call the hormonal continuum, starting with the process of hormone changes called *perimenopause*, a period of time leading up to menopause, when your period ceases for good. This is a major life shift for all women and one that brings up so many questions, both medical (Do I need hormone replacement therapy? Do I need to worry about bone density? Will these hot flashes ever end?) and personal (What does it mean to be a menopausal woman in our youth-obsessed culture?).

Following our trip, I went down the research rabbit hole, reading every bit of research on aging, perimenopause, and menopause that I could, searching for any way to turn back the clock, anything that would keep others from seeing me as "old."

Needless to say, my frenzied obsession with staying young was futile and just left me feeling more drained and hopeless than I did on that trail in Peru. But after spending some quality time with the medical literature—and sifting through my own complex feelings about aging—I came to an epiphany. I didn't want to be forever young; rather, I wanted to live as long as possible while still being able to do the things I enjoyed the most. Getting older and entering perimenopause do not mean I lose my value as a woman, not by a long shot. In fact, I believe the best is yet to come—for me and for you.

What I discovered in my newfound mission to optimize my health and longevity is that small changes to diet and lifestyle have profound impacts on our hormone health, risk of disease, and life span, meaning that each of us has the power to truly shape the trajectory of our lives. I have immense satisfaction knowing that the choices I make each day and the healthy habits I've developed will allow me to continue going on backpacking trips with my family for decades to come. Yes, even when I am truly an old lady. And rather than shy away in embarrassment at my age, I choose to be proud of my achievements and the life I've built.

UNDERSTANDING THE
HORMONAL CONTINUUM

Getting older is inevitable, as are going through hormone changes that lead to perimenopause, menopause, and ultimately postmenopause, a process I call the *hormonal continuum*. At some point, the hormones you've come to know and understand over the past few decades of your fertile years (when most women experience a period every 28 days or so, except when they are pregnant) begin to shift, leading ultimately to menopause—a time marked by one year without a period—and then a new life postmenopause. This doesn't happen overnight. And even though it's natural to fear these changes—after all, society makes them sound really unpleasant, from hot flashes to "menopause weight gain," disrupted sleep, and even thinning hair—I promise you that you don't have to experience your mother's menopause! We cannot stop the clock, but we can most definitely make choices today that will create better tomorrows. Not only can we stop aging poorly, but we can make choices that will help us discover new gifts and make these years the best.

Not long ago, hardly anyone was talking about menopause—women were having quiet conversations with their doctors, but it was just not discussed in an open or public way. Now the conversation has opened, but there's still a scarcity of information around it, especially about perimenopause, the time of transition that precedes menopause when you experience some very intense hormonal fluctuations. These fluctuations bring with them body-wide changes that are mystifying, confusing, frustrating, and destabilizing if you don't know what to expect. To put it bluntly, they make your health feel like a train wreck. What's going on and how did it get so off the rails? More important, what can you do about it?

Until very recently, the aging woman and discussions of perimenopause were an obscure, almost taboo topic that no one online wanted to touch. After all, we spent very little time talking about menopause and exactly no time on perimenopause in medical school. For the longest time, social media on women's health was largely focused on pregnancy and not much else. However, in the past couple of years, women have started asking, "Hey, is this normal? I'm only forty-five! There's no way I'm near menopause." The more women speak up about their experiences and ask questions about their journey on the hormonal continuum, the more normalized discussions of perimenopause become, and the more evidence-based health information becomes available to the people who need it most. Advice from social media is not the same as a medical opinion from your doctor, but informational videos, such as the content I post, may help people see themselves on the hormonal continuum and prompt them to seek solutions for their symptoms.

In the coming pages, I'll shed light on the answers to these questions and more. I'll give you the clarity you deserve and spotlight the misinformation around perimenopause and menopause that has interfered with your ability to feel your best. We'll investigate questionable "cures" for what you're dealing with. Together, we'll talk about how you can use one of the most basic and effective treatments—nutrition—to get back on the path to extraordinary health. The primary thrust of my program is lifestyle focused because I wholeheartedly believe that lifestyle changes like nutrition and exercise modifications can make a profound difference in how you experience perimenopause and menopause, and I've seen this proven time and time again with me and my patients. But I will also tell you everything you need to know to navigate the medical side of these hormone changes, including how to talk to your doctor and demystifying hormone replacement therapy. Knowledge is key to not only understanding the changes taking place in your body but to doing something about them. I recognize this, which is why I'm on a mission to help you understand what your body is going through, make necessary lifestyle changes, and discover the path that is right for you.

Who am I to write this book, other than a woman going through this myself? I'm a double-board-certified doctor of medicine, specializing in allergy/immunology and internal medicine, and I've spent more than two decades as a nutrition specialist, having trained at the Cornell University Division of Nutritional Sciences. In medical school, I completed two years of research, studying women's hormones and how they affect the immune system, which sparked my interest in the women's health and wellness space. I've worked one-on-one with thousands and thousands of women in my medical practice. I've written two bestselling books on issues near and dear to women—hunger and fatigue—called *I'm So Effing Hungry* and *I'm So Effing Tired*. Whenever I see a patient in her late thirties, forties, or fifties, I know to ask her about symptoms related to perimenopause and menopause, two critical transitions in her life—symptoms like hot flashes, vaginal dryness, mood swings, anxiety, weight gain, memory problems, and others. The more I talk to women, the more I realize they are ignored, confused, and anxious about what is happening to their bodies. Many are discouraged by their current circumstances and unable to resolve symptoms that have destabilized their lives. Not only that, but they are also getting short shrift on proper health care from the medical community.

My goal, especially when it comes to nutrition and lifestyle, is to empower you to go through stages of life with confidence and clarity, and to finally understand the hormonal continuum—a three-stage series of physical and emotional changes every woman goes through. Perimenopause is the first of the three stages women enter; followed by menopause, when your menstrual periods cease; then postmenopause, which continues toward the end of a woman's natural life. All three stages involve massive hormonal changes that affect virtually every organ, from the skin to the bones to the brain.

These changes usher in a roller coaster of physical and emotional symptoms, incited by dramatic shifts in hormones. We'll look closely at how to manage and alleviate these symptoms through natural and accessible means, and I believe you will be encouraged by what you learn and apply here. This book is an invitation into that experience.

With so many women moving through this continuum—over one billion in 2025[1]—I'm convinced that we need a new and different set of tools to help women not only manage their debilitating symptoms but live their fullest lives.

My approach to health and to women's issues is more holistic than that of many mainstream doctors. I've always felt like Western medicine hasn't paid enough attention to the contribution of diet to health, the prevention of disease, and now to the management of perimenopause, menopause, and postmenopause—all of which are obvious connections to me.

In so many cases, women I've seen have great lives and much to be grateful for—they have fulfilling careers and loving families, and make amazing contributions to their communities. But unless she's prepared for them, a woman can hold on for only so long before perimenopausal and menopausal symptoms rock that kind of world to pieces with unpleasant symptoms like disrupted sleep and unexpected weight gain. Women want to feel good again, and something must be done! The place to start is the food you eat.

THE POWER OF GOOD NUTRITION

My big epiphany came from an unlikely source: my 16-year-old son. Days before his sixteenth birthday, he slipped in the bathroom and broke his jaw. His jaw had to be wired shut to heal, and he was only allowed to "eat" thin liquids. Even smoothies had to be strained, removing any fiber, seeds, or pulp. He was ravenous but could not eat. Days went by on just Gatorade and juice. On day 3 (I will explain the relevance of this later) he turned from an energetic, happy-go-lucky kid into a child who was tired, lethargic, moody, and unmotivated—he lacked any get-up-and-go to do anything, from school activities to sports.

After about 4 weeks, he transitioned to soft food, and we started giving him special soft foods with fiber, protein, healthy fats, and micronutrients. After several days of eating this more expanded diet, the transformation was miraculous. My son was back—he was once again energetic, happy, and motivated.

This is the power of nutrition.

In my previous books, I've written extensively about the importance of our gut health, or microbiome. Witnessing my son's transformation was further proof that we are so connected to our gut when it comes to our mood, cravings, and hormonal balance. It made me even more adamant and passionate about teaching this to my family, patients, and to you. Once you understand the power of nutrition and lifestyle choices to influence your overall feeling of confidence, energy, and motivation, the game changes.

Better nutrition is a framework for not only a better body but also a better brain and longer life. Traditionally, menopause symptoms were addressed with pharmaceutical treatments such as hormone therapy and antidepressants, which are great and can be truly life-changing in many cases. But I don't think that's where we need to start. For one, you'll be experiencing hormone changes before you might be ready for menopausal hormone therapy (MHT). But more important, nutrition is truly the foundation of it all.

Focusing on nutritional needs of women in perimenopause and menopause, I came up with a plan to help women sail through these transitions and experience a massive transformation in their health. I knew I had to share it with as many women as I could, and I began to do so in my practice and online. Jennifer, a 45-year-old mother who follows me on Instagram, reached out and said, "I'm so confused about my hormones. I was taught about puberty and pregnancy, but no one talked to me about perimenopause." She asked for resources on everything she needed to know about perimenopause, a sort of primer that she could use not only for herself but to pass along to her friends and even her teen daughter. That got me thinking. Jennifer is one of countless women all over the world who knows her body is changing but is not sure what that means for her health and hormones. I kept researching, posting, and interacting with women to learn more about their experiences. This book is the culmination of my efforts to help women like Jennifer. I've already seen this plan work for thousands of women, and I believe it can change anyone's experiences through perimenopause, menopause, and postmenopause for the better. Welcome to the Shah Protocol.

THE SHAH PROTOCOL IS FOR YOU

Nutrition should be the first thing discussed in perimenopause, yet it rarely is, and women are left to suffer without knowing this solution. Even on the North American Menopause Society (NAMS) website and in their informative materials, there is no section on food or nutrition, although there is a section on supplements. We desperately need a more open discussion around nutrition for midlife. It would benefit women everywhere.

Good news: I am here to be your guide through this journey. I can't say it enough or in too many ways: The right food is the key to your experience; it will determine the amount of healthy time you spend in this transition and beyond. My plan is based on several underlying principles that I will lay out in detail throughout this book. But here is the short version: Our hormones, immune system, gut, and metabolism go way out of kilter during the menopause transition, with various resulting symptoms.

The key to course-correcting is to alter your nutrition. I promise you: It can have a transformative effect. The right diet can support your hormones and even mitigate the need for hormone therapy during perimenopause and after. (Please know that if you're currently on some kind of hormone medication, I'm not recommending that you drop it cold turkey because of this book. The advice I'm sharing is complementary with HT, and you should always talk to your doctor before discontinuing any medication or adjusting dosages.)

Your body goes through numerous changes as you move further down the hormonal continuum. Because of those changes, you require more of certain nutrients, including protein, fiber, probiotics, and various vitamins and minerals—all of which are obtainable from food. Eating the right hormone-supporting foods that are rich in fiber, taking probiotics, and adding fermented foods, among other strategies, can help realign your changing system. Food has an enormous ability to nourish your body during these stages, and good nutrition is associated with the reduction and relief of symptoms and dramatic decreases in the risk of most serious diseases, from heart disease to depression to osteoporosis to problems in cognition. It may even boost your longevity. The choices you make each day about how you eat and how you live can make a huge difference in your quality of life and set the stage for your long-term health.

The other part of my nutrition framework is not just what you eat but *when* you eat. Our bodies are designed to run perfectly and work and rest right on time, thanks to our natural *circadian rhythm*—the internal clock that regulates our sleep-wake cycle and repeats every 24 hours. Eating according to this rhythm—which I call *circadian fasting*—helps get you off this hormonal roller coaster and promotes much-improved long-term health.

Which brings us to this book. It reshuffles food and nutrition to the top of the priority list as you go through this transition and beyond. You will learn to eat to beat your symptoms—and more.

For example, you'll increase certain fiber-rich, prebiotic vegetables, along with healthy proteins, quality plant-based fats, and fermented foods. The diet is predominantly plant-based, as well as gluten-free and dairy-free, but you can certainly add certain other high-quality foods as long as you can tolerate them. A diet that is very high in plant foods helps guard against weight gain, even for women who are already struggling with being overweight. Did you know that the prevalence of obesity has almost tripled since 1975?[2] Excess weight amplifies symptoms, which is why intervention should always start with nutrition. The key is to focus on increasing the amount and diversity of these foods and avoid ultra-processed foods whenever possible to give yourself the best chance for a healthy, vital mind and body.

HOW THE SHAH PROTOCOL WORKS

The Shah Protocol is the nutrition and lifestyle framework I use in my practice and recommend during speaking engagements and on social media. While I have shared the general premise of the protocol online, this book will be much more detailed, more nuanced, and more supportive. I will walk you through the entire protocol, helping you transition into this new way of eating, thinking, and being and providing you with recipes to get you started. Even though the protocol seems simple, I assure you that it will transform your life. To create the plan, I took the science-backed changes that made the largest impact on my patients and distilled them into a robust protocol.

The Shah Protocol is a 7-day plan designed to jump-start your health and work with your changing hormones through accessible changes to your diet, exercise, and lifestyle choices. Seven days is enough time to notice changes in the gut and quality of sleep. After that, you simply repeat the protocol, personalizing it to your food preferences, schedule, and overall lifestyle. The plan is designed to be flexible and comprises small changes that are easy to adopt and convert to long-term habits—this isn't boot camp. I want you to think of this as a lifestyle revision plan rather than a quick fix. If you revert to your former way of eating, the symptoms will return. I want you to have consistency with this plan and full symptom relief. Your body's needs are changing as your hormones change, but the Shah Protocol is there to keep you healthy and thriving at any stage of life.

You'll also learn several mind-blowing facts and how to act with *Quick Pauses,* which show you what foods and techniques you can use in the moment for quick symptom relief. These pauses are like your SOS emergency relief when you're dealing with symptoms that can be disruptive to daily life. Most of the time, there are things you can do to offer you relief right away. We need tools like this to stop symptoms in their tracks so we can make the most of every minute of every day. I'm here to give them to you.

There's a lot of noise out there and conflicting—even debilitating—advice. This book tunes out all the distractions and misinformation and offers a much simpler and easy-to-understand plan that can elevate your lifestyle and health to the next level. When you center your focus especially on nutrition, you can eliminate the confusion caused by idle trends, quick-fix products, and unsubstantiated hype.

I've also woven in the experiences and successes of real women, so you won't feel alone but empowered, and I share lots of interesting studies and research throughout. These are women who were cranky, depressed, worn-out, plagued with brain fog and low libido, having hot flashes and night sweats, aching with migraines and more, who became renewed, empowered, and transformed after following this protocol. One by one, they experienced revitalized well-being while going through one of the most challenging times of their lives. Their experiences have been astonishing, and I know they will inspire you.

After you've made the simple nutritional changes I recommend, expect the following:

- Improved mood and less anxiety
- Better sleep
- Healthy digestion
- Higher libido
- Sharper thinking
- Diminished hot flashes and night sweats
- A fitter figure, including around your waist
- Greater energy, less fatigue
- And more

Your body is changing, cycling through completely normal phases of life that we all journey through. You cannot control how your hormones change, but you can control how you experience it. With the protocol and tools in this book, you have the power to reframe menopause as an opportunity not a curse.

YES, THIS BOOK WILL HELP YOU NOW

Most of my patients reach a point of true anxiety and even desperation when their hormones start to shift with perimenopause. Don't panic! This book is here for you. In these pages, I will share:

- A detailed explanation of the hormone continuum that demystifies the changes your body is going through
- An explanation of the transition to perimenopause and menopause and its effect on your mood, weight, brain, sleep, and more
- Common perimenopausal, menopausal, and postmenopausal symptoms and how to evaluate their severity
- How this transition alters your gut and immune system and what to do about it
- The clear indications for hormone therapy, along with how HT works, what options you have, and how to talk to your doctor if you think you may need additional support
- A nutritional strategy that provides you with a framework for every day, every meal, regardless of your diet, budget, or location. (It uses real food, accessible from your supermarket, that's easy to prepare.)
- Seventy-seven delicious recipes to get you started
- Supplements that can potentially help relieve symptoms. (Although supplements are not equivalent to whole foods, which come with their synergistic mix of nutrients, not to mention health-building phytochemicals, supplements can help pave the way to your best physical and mental self. You won't be popping a lot of supplements, but there are a few well-studied

ones that are beneficial on your journey, including vitamin D, magnesium, and omega-3s. I'll give you lots of guidance about what to take and how.)

- Science-supported lifestyle strategies to help you ease the transition. (While nutritional changes are potent tools, there's a broader spectrum of lifestyle factors that can support you or even empower you to be your best self. These include breathing exercises, stress-relieving science, ways to boost your sleep quality, and exercise. For example, incorporating strength training is a way to tackle the natural reduction of muscle mass during perimenopause that leads to weaker bones, injury, and a slower metabolism.)

Most important, I hope to empower you and make you realize that the best is yet to come. You are a badass, and my job is merely to help you realize that.

We have 4,000 weeks of life on this earth if we're lucky. As women, nearly half of our weeks are spent living in various states of transition. Let's make all those weeks the healthiest, most fulfilling and meaningful that we can. And let's start now.

PART I

Much Ado About (Peri)Menopause

CHAPTER 1

The Hormone Continuum

I WAS FORTY-THREE WHEN I FIRST began feeling weird, kind of wonky. I had no idea what was happening," says Linda. "I started getting hot flashes, gaining weight, and feeling unusually irritable. I just figured I was getting older and my body was slipping downhill."

"Linda" is one of many women I work with. Like her, around your late thirties to forties, you might start experiencing signs that something's off with your body. Perhaps you're more tired than usual, overreacting to what should be small conflicts, or having irregular cycles with heavier or lighter periods. Maybe you're starting to experience vaginal dryness, and intercourse is painful. You're wondering if there's something wrong with you, even though these changes seem subtle.

As jarring as these realizations can be, it's all perfectly normal. As women, our lives go through big transitions (whereas men's do not), moving from our childbearing years that start with puberty and progressing into our infertile years. We live life on a continuum with different stages—*perimenopause, menopause,* and *postmenopause.*

None of these stages is just a medical condition; each is a journey that tests your resilience, patience, and ability to adapt. They teach you how to listen to your body, prioritize your health, and embrace the support of those around you.

Though challenging, this journey can be enlightening, revealing strengths you never knew you had and giving you a deeper compassion for other women's experiences. It's why I strongly believe that your thirties, forties, fifties, and beyond can be the best years of your life. With all its trials and tribulations, each stage is not just an end but a beginning, a new chapter that holds the promise of wisdom, growth, and renewed vitality.

HORMONAL UPHEAVAL

Physically, the hormonal continuum is all about sex hormones— mainly estrogen, progesterone, and to some extent testosterone. Our sex hormones are very complex. From puberty to postmenopause, they're responsible for the many hormonal, physical, and mental changes that happen over the span of a lifetime. These hormones help regulate reproductive function, sexual performance, and libido. But they are also involved in many other aspects of health, including bone and muscle strength, skin integrity, and mood, to name just a few. Because estrogen, progesterone, and testosterone are so inter-connected with the rest of the body, it's no surprise that if we alter their delicate balance, we can experience a wide range of symptoms.

Estrogen

Estrogen is what makes us uniquely female, thank you very much, although men have a minute amount of this hormone as well. It's pivotal in our sexual development, and along with progesterone, it regulates the entire reproductive system throughout our lives. It's hard to decide what level of estrogen is normal—this varies widely among women and throughout the course of their monthly cycle. What's more important is the balance of estrogen to progesterone. They work together as a team.

Apart from its role in menstruation, estrogen has other duties you might not be aware of, including protecting bone health and cardiovascular health, and stabilizing your mood. This is because there are estrogen receptors everywhere in the body, allowing this hormone to call the shots on a wide variety of bodily functions. Receptors work sort of like locks, while the substances binding to them—in this case, estrogen—are the keys to those locks. The more estrogen receptors, the more estrogen there is to access cells and do its work. Estrogen keeps your skin soft, supple, and youthful. It also protects against cardiovascular disease and fights chronic inflammation, which occurs when your body's natural immune-fighting power goes into overdrive and can damage organs.

Estrogen also plays a role in regulating your weight. With perimenopause, estrogen levels fall off naturally, but in doing so, it may create hormonal fluctuations. In response, your body tries to protect itself by storing fat—especially around your waist (estrogen exists in fat tissue, too). Because fat tissue is a source of estrogen, your body clings to it relentlessly as your estrogen levels continue to fluctuate. This is one reason why we tend to gain weight during perimenopause and menopause or after a hysterectomy. Estrogen also influences appetite, which explains why you may be feeling hungrier and eating more than usual. But if you can maintain a healthy weight and create healthy levels of estrogen, not too high or too low, you lower your risk of weight gain throughout the continuum. My protocol is designed to help you do just that.

Estrogen is truly one of the body's star players. Once it's released, it travels through the bloodstream to where it's needed; from there, this hormone binds to an estrogen receptor, a type of protein, from which it supports all kinds of processes throughout the body. It protects memory, helps us sleep better, and keeps our joints mobile and healthy.

Quick Pause: Support Estrogen Levels with a Sniff

Essential oils are concentrated plant extracts and may be just the magic you need for hormonal support. Besides smelling great, they may also support estrogen production throughout the menopausal continuum, especially during perimenopause.

The authors of a study reported in *Neuroendocrinology Letters* in 2017 said this: "It has long been recognized that some essential oils have the efficacy of alleviating menopausal symptoms. On the basis of this, it is possible that these essential oils have the potency to facilitate estrogen secretion in women."[1]

These researchers went to work, discovering that sniffing the aroma of certain essential oils increased the production of estrogen in women's salivary glands. Although most estrogen is made in the ovaries, some is manufactured in these glands. In fact, this is why you can collect a saliva sample to check your estrogen levels.

The researchers tested ten different essential oils, and all were found to boost estrogen:

Clary sage. This oil contains a substance called sclareol, known to act like estrogen in the body. For this reason, clary sage oil is believed to be helpful in reducing certain symptoms of menopause. Some research hints that clary sage oil diluted in a carrier oil such as olive oil or coconut oil and rubbed on the bottoms of your feet can relieve hot flashes.[2]

Frankincense. Known as the "king of oils," frankincense can help reduce inflammation, boost mood, and improve sleep.

Geranium. This essential oil is used to reduce inflammation, ease anxiety, and support hormone production.

Lavender. This popular oil can ease stress, reduce pain, and improve sleep. Before the discovery of antiseptics, lavender was used as a sanitizing agent in hospitals.

Jasmine absolute. Getting just a whiff of this essential oil is uplifting. It has been used to fight depression and is considered an aphrodisiac.

Neroli. This versatile essential oil is beneficial for several conditions, including depression, anxiety, high blood pressure, and various menopausal symptoms.

Rose otto. This oil has anti-aging and anti-stress properties and is considered a libido booster. It is also recommended for general hormone support.

Ylang ylang. Lots of benefits come from ylang ylang: better mood, less anxiety, and lower blood pressure.

Chamomile–orange and Roman. All varieties of chamomile essential oil reap benefits because they are calming and soothing to the central nervous system. Both versions are thought to relieve perimenopausal symptoms.

How to use essential oils: You can diffuse them into the air with a diffuser, which is a type of aromatherapy. Or simply take a deep whiff of the aroma after opening the bottle. Try placing a few drops of the essential oil on a cotton ball and breathe in the aroma as it disperses. Another technique is to drop a bit of the essential oil into a bowl of hot water. Position your head over the bowl, place a towel over your head, and breathe in the steam.

Progesterone

Estrogen and progesterone work as a team of hormones to regulate bodily processes, namely menstruation. After you ovulate, estrogen levels dip slightly, and progesterone is released. This hormone is produced by a temporary gland called the *corpus leteum* in your ovaries and peaks at about day 21 of your cycle. It's also produced in adrenal glands as well as the placenta. Progesterone thickens the lining of your uterus so that the fertilized egg can implant. It also helps secrete nutrients that nourish the newly fertilized egg. During pregnancy, your progesterone levels continue to rise until your baby is born. After birth, your progesterone levels drop back to their pre-pregnancy averages.

As you progress along the continuum into perimenopause, your periods are more sporadic and infrequent. Eventually the production of progesterone is much lower. This reduced level of progesterone is what triggers many perimenopausal symptoms. Progesterone is known as the calming hormone, and if you're struggling with anxiety, irritability, and mood swings, that's possibly a progesterone imbalance making you feel crazy. Many women in perimenopause and menopause who suffer from mood-related issues and intense physical symptoms associated with the natural decline of estrogen and progesterone may be prescribed estrogen progesterone hormone therapy (EPT), or combination therapy, by their OB-GYN to stabilize their hormone-related symptoms. For more information on hormone therapies, visit chapter 3.

Testosterone

Estrogen and progesterone aren't the only players here. Nor are they the only ones in short supply during these stages; testosterone is, too. Although testosterone is typically thought of as only a male hormone, women make it to a lesser degree in our ovaries and adrenals. It keeps our hair and skin healthy, makes us excited for sex, gives us good muscle tone, and keeps our bones strong. It also helps with memory and focus, as well as keeping us energetic.

When testosterone levels are low, a lot of things take a turn for the worse. We have thinning hair and dry skin. Intercourse is painful because of dryness (not to mention loss of our sex drive), and we can lose muscle tone, feel depressed, and have depleted energy.

A 2022 review published in the *International Journal of Impotence Research* emphasized: "Testosterone is a vital hormone in women in maintaining sexual health and function" after menopause.[3] Yet until recently, standard menopause care mostly ignored testosterone. If you aren't sold on the idea of taking a hormone you've been told all your life is for men, don't worry; there are foods and exercises you can use to naturally boost testosterone and stay wonderfully feminine.

THE STAGES OF THE
HORMONAL CONTINUUM

We hear a lot about menopause, but the truth is there is not one stage or one moment that defines this period for women. Let's find out more about these stages of the continuum.

Premenopause

Most of my team comprises women in their twenties, and I've been shocked by their rapt curiosity surrounding the hormonal continuum and the strategies they can incorporate into their lives to make transitions through life easier. While many on my team are nowhere near menopause, they've taken a deep interest in how to change their diet and lifestyle to be ahead of the game.

I can guarantee that having a proper diet and healthy lifestyle in your twenties and thirties will make your perimenopause symptoms much more pleasant or even nonexistent. Read that again because it's absolutely true. If you have your diet, exercise, and lifestyle dialed in, you're not going to have a difficult hormonal transition reflective of the horror stories we hear about aging. Our diet and lifestyle choices influence every process within the body, which includes hormonal changes we go through as we get older.

A strong gut and smart lifestyle will keep you clear-minded and energized as your hormones change. Consider the late luteal phase of your cycle, the week before your period, for example. It's the week where you experience premenstrual syndrome (PMS) most intensely, your progesterone and estrogen levels drop, and you experience headaches, bloating, nausea, and more. You may recall that these are some of the same symptoms as in perimenopause.

Since the late luteal phase of your cycle is something of a mini perimenopause, you can likely guess where I'm going with this. Not only will having your nutrition and exercise dialed in help you ease into perimenopause, but it will also help you manage the symptoms you experience during menstruation.[4] Now, this isn't to say that your cramping, bloating, nausea, and other symptoms will disappear leading up to and during your period; however, optimizing your gut-brain-hormone connection while you're young and still having regular cycles will serve to minimize the discomforts of your period naturally.

Okay, so maybe you've already begun your journey into perimenopause and you're thinking, "It's a little late for that now." It isn't. It is never too late to make small changes to your lifestyle that will have a substantial impact on your longevity and hormonal health. Further, if you're a mother with daughters or you're close with young women in your life, share with them what you now know! Knowledge is power no matter where you are on the hormonal continuum.

I don't claim to have all the answers, but I can tell you that I know infinitely more about my body now than I did when I was 20. While I thought I knew everything back then, I most certainly didn't. If only I had had someone in my life to clue me in to what was yet to come: the struggles, the burnout, the triumph, the beauty, and the many changes I would later experience.

When I'm thinking about why I do what I do, why I've built this platform and community for women's health, I often picture my younger self and how much I didn't know. There are so many women out there who are just like my 20-year-old self, and I do all this so that they may have an easier transition and be at peace with themselves in their ever-changing body. All of us deserve the power of knowing our bodies and how to best care for them, and that starts by developing constructive lifestyle habits and practicing them over time, whether that be in our twenties, thirties, forties, or beyond.

Perimenopause

Perimenopause is the stage where you begin to notice some of the more common symptoms of menopause (we'll go over these in the next chapter). It's when a dwindling ovarian reserve begins to take its toll on your body, causing drastic fluctuations in estrogen and progesterone.

Let's back up a second. An infant is born with all the eggs they will ever have—usually between one and two million. Eggs are not produced over the course of a woman's life; instead they decline steadily. At puberty, the number of eggs will have decreased to between 300,000 and 400,000; the number then decreases by 1,000 each month after the first menstrual period. During your reproductive years, each month your pituitary gland sends a signal of follicle-stimulating hormone (FSH) to your ovaries, telling the immature eggs there to start to grow. As this happens, more estrogen and progesterone are made. Then a hormone called *inhibin B* turns off a switch that stops the pituitary gland from producing more FSH. At this point, one ovary releases a mature egg, and if there is sperm to meet it, conception is possible. If not, then your progesterone levels drop, and you have a period.

Fertility begins to decline during your thirties, and you'll have less than 10 percent of your egg reserve by age 40. Then comes perimenopause, and this whole scenario changes. The pituitary gland still dispatches FSH to stimulate your ovaries to produce more estrogen. Your ovaries are still releasing eggs but not every month like before, and their quality and supply diminish.

So, in perimenopause, your body reacts in different ways to these changing signals. No longer is it used to working with its "normal" pattern of estrogen levels, which are now sputtering wildly. It's no wonder you're experiencing symptoms. Like most grand adventures, the ride can be a little bumpy at first.

When your ovarian reserve reaches roughly 25,000 eggs, voilà, you've entered perimenopause—the on-ramp to menopause that generally happens to many of us in our forties. The average age for perimenopause to start is 45, although around one in one hundred women experience it just before 40 and some as early as their twenties and early thirties. It is a natural stage of your life that can last up to fifteen to twenty years. Unless you know it's around the corner, perimenopause can sneak up on you.

There are two stages of perimenopause, sometimes called "early transition" and "late transition." During the early transition, your cycles are mostly regular but may go from heavy to light, light to heavy, sometimes with spotting, sometimes with flooding. These irregularities become more frequent as you enter the late transition, and everyone who has periods will one day stop having them.

The intensity of many other symptoms ramps up, too, as you wade further into perimenopause and closer to menopause. Women in the late transition, for example, are more likely to develop major depression. Further, studies show that women with low levels of anxiety tend to become highly anxious as they progress through the transition. Tragically, depression and anxiety make perimenopausal women more prone to suicide. According to a 2023 study in *BJPsych Bulletin*, the highest rates of suicide in women in England and Wales are seen in the 45-to-49-year-old age group (7.8 per 100,000 in 2021).[5] It's no coincidence that these age-group stats reflect the transitional time leading up to menopause.

I also read a survey of four thousand women revealing that one in ten had quit their jobs and 14 percent had reduced their working hours because of debilitating symptoms connected to these transitional phases of their lives.[6] Being a working mom like so many women across the nation, I was shocked by these statistics, especially since there are more women in the workforce than ever before and they need the income.

Confusingly, perimenopausal symptoms may not start out with the obvious ones such as hot flashes or night sweats. They may be mental: feeling anxious, moody, or irritable. If you have changes in your period and any of the following signs, it could be hormonal:

- exhaustion
- irregular periods
- inability to fall asleep
- weight gain
- gut problems
- dry skin
- hair loss
- migraines

Some may be embarrassing to bring up: low libido, vaginal dryness, or pain during intercourse.

Why are such things happening? It's easy to understand, really. Remember, with perimenopause, you're in the final years of your reproductive life. The World Health Organization (WHO) estimates that women aged 40 to 44 have a fertility rate of 10 percent; 45 to 49, 2 percent; and women over the age of 50 have low fertility rates, but not 0 percent.[7] While these estimates are not perfect, they give us a rough idea of how fertility declines as we progress into perimenopause and menopause. Rather than ballpark your fertility based on age alone, if tracking fertility is something that's important to you, researchers recommend the Stages of Reproductive Aging Workshop (STRAW), which factors in length of menstrual periods, cycle variability, and your hormones to determine your fertility status.[8] You can use electronic hormone monitors or urinary assay sticks (in addition to consulting your doctor) to help track your cycle and fertility if you're trying to get pregnant in your forties but worry about when you will enter menopause. Naturally, production of the hormones estrogen and progesterone bounces around during perimenopause, with unpredictable fluctuations in levels that can affect the entire body: hot flashes, moodiness, weight gain (especially around the belly), brain fog, migraines, vaginal dryness, sleeplessness, among others. But sometimes not. You may never feel any of these symptoms because here's the bottom line: *All women are different.*

This is partly because our psychosocial experience influences our physical and mental experiences. Your perimenopause will be influenced by everything from your quality of life; levels of stress; physical health, including any conditions you might have such as diabetes; and mental status, including a history of depression, anxiety, and other mood disorders.

Racial and ethnic differences also influence your experience. The Study of Women's Health Across the Nation (SWAN), for example, found that African American women in perimenopause may have more frequent symptoms such as hot flashes and night sweats compared with other racial groups.[9] It's been reported that their symptoms are also more painful and cause more discomfort—and no one is sure why.

Whatever our symptoms, nearly 90 percent of perimenopausal women trudge into their doctors' offices complaining of symptoms and desperately wanting relief.[10] Understanding and managing symptoms are huge challenges for us.

Because perimenopausal and menopausal symptoms are mostly nonspecific, general practitioners have received little or no training on how to deal with them; therefore, our symptoms are largely marginalized and dismissed. Perimenopause is not an illness, either— it's a natural stage of life—and most physicians are trained to treat only illnesses. My OB-GYN friends have even said that perimenopause was not made to be a part of their medical education beyond brief mention. The unique experiences of women going through perimenopause are often trivialized by the conventional medical community.

Take the case of Melissa, a busy writer juggling several projects at once who went into perimenopause knowing nothing about it or that it even had a name. She was 45 when severe migraines hit. They were relentless, not letting up for days on end, to the point where she had to lie down in the middle of the day due to the crushing pain. Desperate, Melissa went to her doctor for help and was prescribed Imitrex, a migraine pain reliever, but it made her feel drowsy and dizzy. Her doctor then ordered a brain scan, which to Melissa was anxiety-provoking both before the scan and then waiting for the results. The thought that she might have a brain tumor was paralyzing and interfered with both her work and home life. Fortunately, the brain scan was clear—no tumors or lesions. The results of follow-up visits to her doctor were also inconclusive. So, what was causing the migraines?

Around the same time, Melissa started having night sweats in which she would wake up drenched in perspiration, no matter what the bedroom temperature. Then, a chance reading of a study reported in *Prevention* mentioned "perimenopause" and how low estrogen levels can trigger debilitating symptoms like the ones she was experiencing.[11] It was finally the validation she had been looking for. The culprit that no doctor had mentioned? Her hormones. They had started to go haywire, spiking and dipping seemingly at random. Melissa realized she was in full-blown perimenopause, a word not in her vocabulary before.

Melissa's story is sadly common. No physician or health care practitioner had mentioned perimenopause or the role that fluctuating hormones played in her newfound discomfort or how to tackle the situation. Eventually and through her own digging, Melissa found that a lot could be done about all this—naturally and holistically— and she was able to reclaim her life.

The very subject of perimenopause has always been taboo because some of its symptoms are embarrassing (like hair loss, vaginal dryness, and painful sex), and it signals that our bodies are aging (who likes to face up to *that*!). Basically, no one has really talked openly about perimenopause.

What's more, there's very little evidence-based information about perimenopause. Despite major advances for women over the past one hundred years—the invention of birth control pills and better screenings for women's health—much of female biology is still woefully neglected by scientific research. There are reasons for this, most notably the historical omission of women from clinical trials, partly because our hormonal cycles were believed to skew results. There's also the fact that some researchers still project results from studies on men onto women, forgetting we are not men! We are different—and not just anatomically. We're different right down to the cellular level, meaning that many of our immune responses, pain threshold, and symptoms (including those that signal a heart attack) may be different from men's. Even most drugs were developed with the male body in mind, even though the side effects on women may be vastly different from men's.

Also, there are very distinct differences between the female and male gut. For one thing, the female colon is longer than the male colon, on average nearly four inches longer. The reason, experts believe, is that this permits better absorption of water during childbearing in order to maintain healthy levels of amniotic fluid and better circulation during pregnancy.

But this extra length in the colon has a downside. It leads to more bloat and constipation than our male counterparts will ever experience. Have you ever heard your husband, boyfriend, or brother complain about being bloated? Probably not!

Perimenopause (and menopause) can greatly disrupt your gut and bowel habits, too. As your hormones change during perimenopause, so does your gut microbiome (the collection of microorganisms that live in the digestive system). Consequences: weight gain, moodiness, poor immunity, and digestive problems, to name just a few. Men don't have to deal with this stuff; it's rarely a factor with them.

Other statistics talk loudly here, too. As reported by the survey group Statista, 44 percent of women worldwide were unaware of perimenopause until they started having symptoms; 46 percent did not expect perimenopause when it hit; 34 percent did not know that there were two phases of this transition; and 46 percent did not feel prepared for what happens next—menopause.[12]

What concerns me, too, are the clever marketing ploys being used by product companies to drive sales rather than offer actual help. The menopause market is projected to reach $24.4 billion by 2030, making it an attractive avenue for new business.[13] Case in point: A couple of well-known actresses are shamelessly plugging menopause supplements that have not been adequately tested, evaluated, or researched.

Perimenopause is an unpredictable and challenging time of life for many of us, yet we are in the prime of our lives and careers. Some of us are even caught in the sandwich generation, in which we are caring for both our kids and our parents. We, our families, and society can't afford to let any of this human potential slip away. It's therefore critical to understand how perimenopause fits into our lives and to anticipate, address, and alleviate the common and not-so-common symptoms that may so dearly affect our quality of life.

Menstrual Irregularities

Those with irregular cycles, whether caused by various forms of birth control or conditions such as polycystic ovary syndrome (PCOS), endometriosis, pelvic inflammatory disease (PID), thyroid disorders, ovary removal, and more may have a difficult time knowing where they fall on the hormonal continuum. For example, birth control in the form of oral contraceptives minimizes the natural peaks and valleys of our hormones and stabilizes them into more even hormonal states, meaning the ways in which menstrual and perimenopausal symptoms present themselves are different than the symptoms someone cycling without birth control experience because the way they experience their hormones in general is more dynamic.

Everyone's journey through perimenopause is unique, and we all experience the hormonal continuum differently, especially for people on birth control or for those with conditions that affect their cycle. Your doctor might check your vitamin D levels and make a comprehensive assessment of your overall health, but even then, it can be difficult to determine when your hormones are in transition. Unfortunately, there isn't a definite biological indicator (yet) that lets us know where we are on the continuum—barring a pregnancy test, but that is a different book entirely.

My favorite thing about the female body is how remarkably diverse we are. Imagine if one hundred women ate the same foods, exercised the same way, and had the same routine. Now realize that no woman would look, behave, or exist in the same way as the next. Health is such an individual and personal thing, and it is both beautiful and confounding that there is no cut-and-dried, one-size-fits-all answer for how to go through life on the continuum.

While everyone's health is unique to themselves and women's health is a multifaceted area of medicine, we cannot let the complexities and nuances of this subject justify the gaps in knowledge surrounding conditions like PCOS or endometriosis. Roughly 5 to 14 percent of all women (yes, that many) experience either PCOS, endometriosis, or both in their reproductive years.[14] And while these conditions are relatively common, we still do not know nearly enough about them and many other conditions that impact reproductive and hormonal health.

Quick Pause: PCOS and the Gut Microbiome

The medical community has a long way to go when it comes to understanding PCOS and other endocrine conditions that impact female reproductive health. Given that PCOS is such a common condition, you would think we would know what causes it, but we don't. Well, it's generally believed that genetics play a role, or weight, yet there isn't conclusive research on this. What we do know is that PCOS causes the overproduction of the male hormone androgen, insulin resistance, inflammation, and potential infertility. In fact, PCOS is one of the leading causes of infertility in women, and most women don't get a diagnosis until after trying (and not succeeding) to become pregnant. PCOS is characterized by irregular periods, increased acne, hair growth, weight gain, and follicle cysts on the ovaries.

Recent research has identified trends in the gut microbiota of women with PCOS. In a 2023 systematic review and meta-analysis compiling findings from 28 studies, researchers concluded that

PCOS is associated with lower diversity of gut bacteria and can alter gut bacteria that influence processes such as metabolism, inflammation, and hormone regulation.[15] More specifically, people with PCOS have a decreased presence of *Lachnospira* and *Prevotella* bacteria in their gut; these bacteria are responsible for digesting fiber and aiding in the production of short-chain fatty acids (SCFAs). People with PCOS also have higher amounts of *Bacteroides, Parabacteroides, Lactobacillus, Fusobacterium, Escherichia,* and *Shigella,* which all indicate a shift toward a pro-inflammatory gut environment.

What does this mean? Well, from what we can conclude based on current research, an inherent symptom (or characteristic) of PCOS is *gut dysbiosis,* or an imbalance in the bacterial makeup and function of the gut microbiome. Someone with PCOS experiences a reduction in SCFAs and bile acid–metabolizing bacteria essential for keeping inflammation at bay.

Okay, so what does that mean? Treatment for PCOS is not as simple as "just lose weight." It is so much more complex than that. Current treatment pathways for PCOS include insulin-sensitizing medications, hormonal birth control (for people not trying to become pregnant), androgen-blocking medications, and lifestyle changes for a healthy diet and body weight. However, these options don't quite get to the deeper issue here, which is gut dysbiosis. A meta-analysis from 2023 on 17 randomized controlled trials (RCTs) with more than one thousand participants found that increasing prebiotic and probiotic intake contributed to improvements in hormonal balance and a decrease in insulin resistance for participants with PCOS.[16]

Research on this topic is ongoing, and further evidence is needed to recommend specific doses or bacterial strains of pre- and probiotics for treating PCOS. However, the results so far are promising. The gut is powerful and can potentially be the key to better treatment options for conditions like PCOS that have significant impacts on menstruation and fertility.

If you've been misdiagnosed or not taken seriously by your doctor, and if you're someone with a condition that impacts your cycles,

I see you, I acknowledge you, and you can rest assured that this book takes you into consideration. In crafting this protocol, my research hinges on the fact that while we may go through these same fundamental stages of hormonal transition, we experience them in ways that are unique to us. The nexus of the Shah Protocol is simply that it's a flexible set of guidelines that can be adapted to anyone, no matter their health conditions and needs. What you need to internalize is that everything gets better when your gut gets better. No matter what you're going through, taking actions that will improve your gut microbiome will have positive ripple effects throughout the body.

Menopause

You've officially hit menopause when you haven't had a menstrual period for one full year (barring any other medical condition or medication that would have an impact on your periods). Your ovaries have stopped producing most of their estrogen and no longer release eggs. Menopause is a typical, expected part of aging that occurs toward the end of a woman's fertile period. The average age of menopause in the United States is 51, and most women can expect to go through menopause between the ages of 45 and 55.

In menopause, you may still experience the same symptoms you had in perimenopause, although some may disappear or ease in severity. Remember Melissa? She recalls, "Menopause was easy for me—a lot easier than perimenopause. My periods stopped, and that was it. Life went on. I had no symptoms, except for vaginal dryness, which was easily resolved with lubricants. Of course, all of our bodies and situations are different, but for me, menopause was freedom."

Hitting menopause is unique for each of us. Some might breeze through it like Melissa, while others find themselves in a long, often bumpy ride, with additional symptoms that require attention. The reality is that 80 percent of women have symptoms—from brain fog to anxiety, mood problems, insomnia, fatigue, vaginal dryness, and stiff joints—and the foreignness of it all prevents many women from asking for help.

Most women think they need to start taking hormones at this point. Maybe. Maybe not. (I'll cover this in detail later.) Once demonized and now back in favor, menopausal hormone therapy (MHT), often incorrectly referred to as hormone replacement therapy (HRT), has been shoved front and center as the number one treatment for both perimenopause and menopause. MHT can be great for some women, but it's not the first line of attack, nor is it appropriate or available for many women, depending on their health and family history. Plus, more and more women are seeking natural remedies for their symptoms and prefer not to take hormones. If you do choose MHT (in collaboration with your doctor), coupling that with the natural remedies and protocol in this book can help mitigate your symptoms for an overall better experience.

And those mood swings that make you hard to live with and want to hurl coffee cups and plates at your family? Like perimenopause, menopause is also a risky time for moodiness and anxiety. One survey of three thousand women who went to their doctors during menopause revealed that 66 percent were offered antidepressants rather than HT.[17] They're told by their doctors, "Oh, you've got mood swings? You're just stressed out. Here's a prescription for Xanax or Lexapro." These drugs are some of the most commonly prescribed drugs in the United States, but the problem is that their side effects—including addiction—often leave much to be desired.

The conversation around menopause is a bit louder than it is around perimenopause, but many women are still unsure what to do about it or how to deal with symptoms. As a result, menopause and its symptoms can be missed or go undiagnosed and thus treated inadequately. We are left alone to cope with disturbing changes in our bodies, unprepared, and without the resources required to feel our very best.

Postmenopause

The day after menopause, you will be declared in postmenopause. Like perimenopause, postmenopause is not talked about much. That's unfortunate because it's a stage of life you're in for a long time (hopefully). If you've had menopausal symptoms, they begin tapering off, and any that remain are usually manageable.

As the body begins to lack estrogen, starting in perimenopause, we see an uptick in free radicals, or reactive oxygen species (ROS). These ROS cause cell damage in the form of oxidated stress and are associated with higher levels of inflammation, which is why they are believed to be a major agency of disease both during and after menopause.

Once in postmenopause, it's important to understand you're now at a bigger risk for conditions like osteoporosis, heart disease, and urinary tract infections. We'll talk more about this throughout, particularly in chapter 9. For example, dwindling estrogen can lead to an imbalance in cholesterol that may increase your risk of cardiovascular disease. Low estrogen levels can also lead to osteoporosis. This is a weakening of the bone tissues, which can increase your risk of fractures. Osteoporosis occurs when your body starts to reabsorb bone cells faster than it can replace them. Your vaginal lining becomes papery thin, leading to all sorts of issues with urinary health.

On the plus side, life in postmenopause offers refreshed potential. If you have older children, they may have moved out of the house and are pursuing their own life dreams. You may have more time to spend on yourself. You could potentially go back to school or take classes in various subjects, volunteer in a meaningful way, or start a business. The possibilities are endless. Alternatively, women are having children later and later in life for a plethora of reasons, and it isn't uncommon to both have young children and be in postmenopause. If you're a mother in postmenopause, you may notice that your baseline for stress is much lower than when you were in your thirties and forties. You may approach parenting with a calmer mind and more measured responses to small stressors that pop up daily as a mother as compared with a mother in her twenties (we'll talk more about the differences in stress across the hormonal continuum in chapters 6 and 7). As a postmenopausal mom, you have tons of life experience that may inform the ways you parent your children and cause you to encounter fewer uncertainties than younger moms, for example. Another benefit to postmenopause: No more worrying about periods, birth control, and surprise pregnancies—something we don't realize takes up so much mental space until it's no longer a weight on our shoulders.

5 Myths and Facts Around Perimenopause and Menopause

When it comes to perimenopause and menopause, there's no shortage of myths and old wives' tales. Let's debunk them together.

Myth #1: During the menopause continuum, your body stops producing hormones.
Fact: As you go through the three stages, the rate of your hormone production decreases but does not stop. The physical and mental changes you'll experience are a result of fluctuations in estrogen and progesterone, not a total drop-off of these hormones. Hormone production never stops entirely.

Myth #2: Nothing can be done to manage symptoms—you just have to power through them.
Fact: Perimenopause and menopause are natural conditions that don't necessarily require medical treatment! However, they can give us trouble. But the good news is that many lifestyle changes can provide relief, as can MHT, if that's appropriate for you (more on that in chapter 3). There are solutions out there—we will talk about them throughout this book. Doing nothing is not an option (see below).

Myth #3: Without hormone therapy, there's nothing I can do to manage my symptoms.
Fact: Hormone therapy can help many women feel better during this continuum, but it's not a cure-all, nor is it a good fit for many women. Fortunately, your symptoms and overall well-being can benefit from holistic approaches. For example:

- Practice relaxation techniques like deep breathing.
- Avoid smoking and vaping.

- Limit your intake of alcohol and caffeine.
- Eat a healthy, plant-focused diet.
- Stay physically active.
- Maintain a healthy weight by shifting your diet to take into account your changing hormones.

Myth #4: My sex life is over.

Fact: It's true that the lower hormone levels that come with the menopausal continuum can impact your sexual responsiveness and change your vaginal tissues. But the fact is that you can stay sexually active, turned on, and in the mood no matter what stage you're in. There are things you can do to help your sexual health during this time, including:

- Use water-based vaginal lubricants during sex to prevent discomfort.
- Apply vaginal moisturizers regularly.
- Talk to your doctor about hormone therapy.
- Have more sex.
- Perform exercises to help strengthen your pelvic floor, as these muscles are involved in orgasm.
- Follow a healthy lifestyle, with hormone-supporting nutrition to keep you energized.

Myth #5: Weight gain is inevitable during menopausal transition.

Fact: Weight gain can be prevented during perimenopause, menopause, and beyond. For all the reasons explained in this chapter, we are unfortunately more likely to gain some weight during this transition due to declining estrogen and a slower metabolism, but it's not inevitable. To counteract the effects of these factors, I recommend that you exercise at least 3 to 5 times a week while following the Shah Protocol.

WHERE ARE YOU ON THE CONTINUUM?

Where you fall on the menopause continuum is difficult to pinpoint, but your health care provider can give you an idea based on your constellation of symptoms and medical history. Lab tests exist but normally aren't used to diagnose the stages. Under certain circumstances, though, your physician may recommend blood tests to check your levels of:

- Follicle-stimulating hormone (FSH) and estrogen, because your levels of these hormones fluctuate then decline as you get closer to, and enter, menopause.
- You can purchase over-the-counter home tests to check FSH levels in your urine. The tests may tell you whether you have elevated FSH levels and might be in perimenopause or menopause. But, because FSH levels fluctuate during your menstrual cycle, home FSH tests can't really pinpoint whether or not you're in perimenopause or menopause.
- Thyroid-stimulating hormone (TSH). Tests can look at levels of TSH and identify underactive thyroid (hypothyroidism), which can cause symptoms similar to those of menopause. A decline in estrogen (so, menopause) can also put you at greater risk of hypothyroidism, further complicating the issue. If you're experiencing changes in energy and weight and you're concerned it may be related to your thyroid, schedule an appointment with your doctor so they can help you determine the next steps.

Quick Pause: We Might Be Able to Test for Menopause Someday Soon

A 2025 cross-sectional study published in *Frontiers in Endocrinology* found that across more than two thousand women subjects, women with elevated small dense low-density lipoprotein cholesterol (sdLDL-C) levels were identified as being postmenopausal.[18] The significance of this study is that it's looking at biomarkers for the menopausal transition, independent of chronological age. The sdLDL-C levels of the subjects increased gradually the further along the hormonal continuum a woman was, and the levels peaked at postmenopause. This means that there is a clear biomarker that can distinguish a premenopausal woman from a postmenopausal woman, without needing to know age or other personal factors. This study did not note any success in differentiating biomarkers among women in premenopause, perimenopause, or menopause, but that's the next logical direction for inquiry into this vein.

Now, there's obviously a need for further research across a much larger subject population, but this study points toward a future where we may one day be able to test patients to see where they are on the hormonal continuum. If we can test for perimenopause, for example, women will no longer have to live through this guessing game of "Are my hot flashes because of menopause or something else?" If I can pinpoint a patient's position on the hormonal continuum, I can better treat her through preventative care rather than retroactively working to correct out-of-control symptoms. The potential there is huge and could revolutionize the menopausal experience forever. Research into this area is forthcoming, and I for one am eager to see what more we can learn about this journey through biomarker analyses.

It's best to rely on your symptoms. They are usually enough to tell you that you've entered the menopausal continuum. If you have concerns about your symptoms and want to know more about them, that's where we're headed next.

CHAPTER 2

No One Told Me There Would Be Days Like This

I T KEPT HAPPENING DAY AFTER day: this unusual tiredness I just couldn't quite seem to shake. Dragging around like this, I was worried about how to keep pace with my work and family life. I'm a busy physician, a nutritionist, author, podcaster, involved in community and social activities, married to a husband I love, and parenting two active, spirited children. I was immersed in the busyness of life, juggling all my personal and professional demands, while feeling frazzled, overstressed, and exhausted. Ironically, I knew all about fatigue; I literally wrote a book about it. But in this situation, I didn't have answers even for myself. This wasn't the same as everyday fatigue that an otherwise healthy person might experience from time to time. It was much more severe, a constant presence in my life.

Worsening my fatigue was the fact that I couldn't sleep through an entire night. No matter what I tried (melatonin, chamomile tea, or deep breathing), I'd wake up at three in the morning, restless, frustrated, and unable to pinpoint any valid reason as to why.

Whatever was happening, it was taxing and like nothing I had ever experienced before. It wasn't just the fatigue and sleeplessness; it was also the brain fuzziness. My memory, once laser sharp, felt frayed and fleeting. Anything involving concentration, multitasking, and organizing—that is, practically everything important— became completely arduous. I'd forget my words midsentence, then trail off without completing a thought. My motivation was off, and I struggled through work. I felt out of control. I was a hot mess and wanted desperately to put this misery behind me. My body was signaling that something was off, but what? Knowing what I know about health and a healthy lifestyle, brushing it off as just over-working myself wasn't going to cut it. Because truth be told, I was entering the menopause continuum, and perimenopause was the on-ramp.

THE MOST COMMON SYMPTOMS ACROSS THE CONTINUUM

The changes taking place in your body can be very destabilizing, with a lot of confusion about the symptoms they bring. These symptoms—brain fog, fatigue, disrupted sleep, memory and attention issues, along with weight gain, hot flashes, dry skin, and diminished sex drive—eat away at your quality of life and leave you feeling pretty helpless, run down, and just generally messed up. While none of these symptoms will vanish overnight, they can be eased, even resolved, with the nutrition and lifestyle choices you'll learn throughout this book. When you're not consumed by symptoms, you have more freedom to focus on the things that truly matter to your future. It's more time to nurture fulfilling relationships, work on your mindset, and invest in your health and happiness. And that's exactly what this is all about.

So many of these choices are now being substantiated in research, I'm happy to report. Study in point: The *Southern Medical Journal* stated in a review article that although hormone therapy (HT) has been the cornerstone of treatment for menopausal symptoms, thanks to recent research findings, women are seeking holistic options that work but aren't as risky.

The researchers are quoted as saying: "Exercise has been shown to help some women with symptoms of hot flashes, as have relaxation techniques and deep breathing. Dietary changes to incorporate whole foods and soy are thought by some to help with menopausal symptoms and are recommended because of a positive impact on heart disease and obesity; soy isoflavones may also help with menopausal symptoms. Botanicals such as black cohosh and red clover have been shown in some studies to decrease severity and frequency of hot flashes."[1] This is just one report of many that offer us encouragement when we need it the most!

You might be wondering: How long are you going to have to deal with this stuff? The answer is not forever in most cases. Some symptoms will disappear when you hit menopause and postmenopause. There is hope!

Coping with symptoms starts with understanding them and how they start. Armed with this knowledge, you'll have a much easier journey through the continuum, with strategies that will keep you healthy and feeling good. Once you get going on the protocol, you won't give your symptoms much thought at all.

PHYSICAL SYMPTOMS

So just what does the continuum feel like? As mentioned in chapter 1, doctors don't usually run tests to determine if you're in perimenopause. They base the diagnosis on a constellation of symptoms. You may have heard of some of these, but not all of them, so let's take a closer look at the most common symptoms.

Hot Flashes

Hot flashes, or "vasomotor symptoms" in medical lingo, are symptoms we talk about the most, probably because they're so common. Recent evidence indicates that hot flashes are experienced by 30 to 70 percent of perimenopausal women.[2] They're marked by intense, sudden increases in body temperature. Caused by hormonal fluctuations, hot flashes can last, on average, for 7.4 years—in some instances, they may last up to 10 years or more. Seventy-five percent of women have up to ten hot flashes a day. Hot flashes and night sweats are often a late-stage manifestation of perimenopause, meaning that many women in their late thirties and early forties may not yet experience them. Not every woman will experience hot flashes, however, but certain situations amplify the possibility: being overweight, smoking, and suffering from anxiety or depression.

Hot flashes may increase the closer you get to menopause, but don't feel discouraged. Change in diet and lifestyle has been shown in studies to delay menopause symptoms, making them more bearable and almost eliminating certain symptoms. For example, one study showed that changing your diet and lifestyle to lose around ten pounds decreases hot flashes by over 30 percent.

Quick Pause: Put Out That Hot Flash Now

Hot flashes are sudden surges of heat, usually in your chest, neck, and face. They are one of the most common symptoms of both perimenopause and menopause. They hit unexpectedly, so you'll want to be prepared to douse them fast. One way is with food!

You'll learn more about hormone-supporting nutrition later in this book, but for now, realize that eating a diet focused on a variety of plant foods keeps hot flashes (and night sweats) to a minimum.

A nine-year study involving more than six thousand women analyzed the foods eaten by participants and how often they had hot flashes. Women who ate lots of fruits and veggies reported fewer hot flashes than women with different eating patterns. The researchers emphasized that the anti–hot flash diets were high in fiber and had a low intake of trans-fatty acids, which are found in many processed foods.[3]

One of the reasons that eating more plants may help with hot flashes is that many plant foods contain compounds called *phytoestrogens*, which have been shown in some studies to help reduce hot flashes by mimicking some of the functions of estrogen in the body. Foods high in phytoestrogens include flaxseeds, soybeans and edamame, dried foods, sesame seeds, garlic, peaches, berries, tofu, and cruciferous veggies such as broccoli, Brussels sprouts, cabbage, and collard greens.

In addition to eating these foods, you may want to ease off certain foods that can aggravate hot flashes. These include very spicy foods and processed foods that are high in added sugar and fat.

Night Sweats

Night sweats are hot flashes that hit during the night. These can be one of the more disruptive symptoms of perimenopause and menopause because they wake you up in the middle of the night from deep sleep, soaked in sweat, and prevent you from falling back to sleep. Night sweats are uncomfortable, annoying, and lead to sleep issues, which can have a tremendous impact on a variety of physiological and mental health factors.

Irregular Periods

Your period becomes more sporadic as you enter perimenopause—that's pretty much a given, thanks to fluctuations in estrogen and progesterone. Irregular periods can mean bleeding that's lighter or heavier than in the past, more or fewer days of bleeding, and longer or shorter cycles. At menopause and after, your periods stop altogether. If you notice your cycle becoming increasingly irregular and infrequent, this is a strong indicator that you are nearing the end of perimenopause and transitioning into menopause.

Weight Changes

You may find your weight climbing or shifting—for no apparent reason—during perimenopause. On average, women will gain twenty-two pounds between ages 40 and 60.[4] Again, the main culprit is declining estrogen levels. One of estrogen's jobs is to deposit fat onto your hips to prepare you for childbirth. But as estrogen and growth hormone levels decline during perimenopause and your metabolism adapts to lower levels of estrogen, fat accumulation shifts from your hips and thighs to your tummy, resulting in a bigger waistline or "meno-belly." If you were pear shaped as a younger woman, you might become more apple shaped as you get older.

Other hormones are involved here, too. One is cortisol, best known as the stress hormone. Historically, cortisol has saved our lives, helping us outrun hungry saber-toothed tigers. However, given that we're in modern times, your body doesn't differentiate between hungry tigers and financial worries and other life stresses, even though one is life-threatening, and the other is stress-provoking but won't kill you. Belly fat contains receptors (little gateways into cells). Under stress, your adrenals churn out cortisol, and this stimulates these belly fat receptors, and more fat makes its way into fat cells around your belly.

You're also losing muscle at greater rates because of declining estrogen and likely being less active. The net effect is a slowdown in your metabolism. Including weight training in your exercise program prevents muscle loss and weight gain. We'll talk more about the benefits of weight training for women in perimenopause and beyond in chapter 8.

A hormonal problem called "insulin resistance" can also contribute to weight gain. This occurs when your insulin receptors begin to not recognize insulin, mostly the result of eating too many sugary meals for too long. The pancreas keeps releasing insulin to help that sugar get into cells, but eventually that production can't keep pace and slows down. This increases insulin levels in your system that can make the body more easily turn calories into fat—even if you're dieting. Chronic stress and abdominal fat can encourage insulin resistance.

Among the other factors I've listed, the quality of diet is probably the strongest determining element for this stage of life. Luckily for you, a huge chunk of this book is focused on nutrition and knowing what your body needs (and doesn't need) to improve your health and live longer.

Breast Tenderness

Caused by erratic hormone levels, sore and tender breasts are often one of the first indicators of perimenopause. The good news? This symptom is among the first to resolve as you get closer to menopause and your hormones become less volatile.

Quick Pause: Best Relief for Breast Tenderness

Your doctor might consider it a trivial symptom, but breast tenderness, or *mastalgia*, is very uncomfortable for many women. Breast tenderness typically presents in your thirties or forties, right around the time you enter perimenopause. This symptom creates anxiety for many women because they think it might be a symptom of breast cancer. Let me assure you, it's not; it's typically a sign of sputtering hormones and a result of normal changes taking place in your breasts, although it is important to keep up with your regular breast exams, including an annual mammogram from age 40 on. If you notice unusual changes of any kind to your breasts and you're unsure whether they are due to hormonal changes or something else, it's best to reach out to your doctor about your concerns to ensure that it isn't in fact breast cancer. All too often women feel as though their health concerns aren't valid or, worse, their concerns are brushed aside and invalidated by someone close to them or a medical professional. If you have even a shred of fear that a change in your breasts is unusual, please contact your doctor.

The quickest, simplest way to resolve breast tenderness—and the most common first-line treatment—is evening primrose oil, a beneficial fat rich in a substance called gamma linolenic acid (GLA), available as an over-the-counter dietary supplement. It provides pretty fast relief, although it's a good idea to take it for 6 months to achieve the full benefits. The usual dosage is 1,000mg, taken 4 times daily, but check with your health care provider about the best dosage for you.

Sleep Issues

Quality sleep is critical to correcting any type of hormonal blockage or decline. Your ability to think, reason, react, and respond will slow if your sleep is disturbed. This can include things like interrupted sleep, poor quality of sleep, or just having trouble falling and staying asleep.

Why does this happen? Perimenopause makes it hard to sleep because of night sweats, changes in mood, stress, poor-quality diet, and of course fluctuations in hormones—specifically estrogen and progesterone. Lower levels of progesterone during perimenopause and menopause really mess up your beauty sleep because this hormone is what helps induce sleep. Throughout the book, I'll touch on this further and introduce several changes you can make to improve your sleep. Even if you don't suffer from sleep issues (yet), it's always good to examine various lifestyle habits and analyze what's either helping or hurting your circadian rhythm.

Fatigue

As I did, you might notice lower energy levels as you move along the hormonal continuum into perimenopause. The reasons? Because of continual changes in hormone levels, other common perimenopausal and menopause symptoms such as poor sleep, the stress of day-to-day life and its responsibilities, and many, many more. You're not alone, though. One study of three hundred women found that just over 85 percent dealt with fatigue during the menopausal transition.[5] While fatigue is a pesky symptom of perimenopause, and we may not even clock it as a symptom at first, there are several ways to combat the severity or negative effects of fatigue through improving your lifestyle habits with a special emphasis on hormone health.

Vaginal Dryness

During midlife, your vagina is not exempt from the symptoms caused by hormonal slowdowns. Before perimenopause, estrogen is around to promote blood flow to the area, providing oxygen and nutrients that build up the tissue, lubricate it naturally, and keep it moist. Those nutrients also feed collagen and elastin production, two proteins responsible for tissue elasticity in the vagina.

But then perimenopause comes around. You might feel like your private parts are shrinking, and you're right. They are. The labia might diminish, and internal vaginal structures flatten and become less flexible. With these changes come irritation and sometimes painful sex. Multiple studies show that, often, women also experience loss of their sex drive and have trouble orgasming as a result of these hormonal shifts.

The technical term for what's happening is *genitourinary syndrome of menopause* (GSM), which is an update to the negative term *vaginal atrophy*. The symptoms of GSM appear relatively early in the transition. Unlike hot flashes and mood changes, which tend to improve over time, vaginal dryness does not get better without specific ongoing treatment and may continue through menopause and beyond. Fortunately, there are strategies that bring enormous relief.

Lower Sex Drive

Rest assured that your sex life doesn't end during perimenopause, and if you've noticed a decrease in your sex drive, it's likely that other perimenopause symptoms are influencing your desire. As I've said, hormonal changes lead to vaginal dryness, which makes intercourse painful. Testosterone keeps you frisky, but now it's so erratic that sometimes you're just not in the mood. Weight gain and shifts in your body shape may affect your self-image in the bedroom. Plus, the energy drain of not getting enough sleep cuts into your bedroom fun. None of this means you must give up on sex altogether, however. There are ways to make you feel good again. You can remain intimate and enjoy sex with your special someone far beyond perimenopause once you learn how to address your symptoms.

Headaches

For many women, migraines and other headaches intensify during perimenopause and can be debilitating. They are at their worst in the beginning of perimenopause, when hormone levels are especially volatile and unpredictable. Fortunately, some women find that their hormone-triggered headaches become less frequent after menopause, once hormone levels have evened out. Such is the case for many pesky perimenopause symptoms, though that doesn't mean symptoms such as migraines or headaches can't persist postmenopause. If you're struggling with migraines at any stage along the hormonal continuum, it's a good idea to communicate these complaints to your doctor, as you may be a candidate for medication.

Joint Pain

When we're younger, we're as nimble and flexible as rubber bands, thanks to estrogen, which keeps our joints lubricated and prevents inflammation. Then along comes perimenopause with its declining estrogen levels—and voilà, our joints start to hurt and may even swell. As our estrogen declines, so, too, does our vitamin D, which then creates a host of aches and pains in our joints at best and osteoporosis at worst. You can help prevent developing chronic joint pain and mitigate these aches through proper nutrition and exercise, though this symptom may never fully dissipate because it's an inevitable side effect of aging for most people.

Muscle Aches

This symptom is a sign of chronic inflammation, which occurs when too many pro-inflammatory catalysts build up in the body due to poor sleep, stress, a bad diet, and so forth. As a result, the body becomes more susceptible to disease and infection. Estrogen is an unsung hero when it comes to fighting chronic inflammation. During perimenopause, however, loss of inflammation-easing estrogen can also contribute to sore muscles. One study found that 71 percent of perimenopausal women experienced musculoskeletal pain.[6] That's most women! We'll go over different strategies you can try to manage painful muscle aches.

Quick Pause: Sprinkle This Spice on Your Food Now

I've been eating the spice turmeric in my foods since childhood because it is the number one seasoning of my native Indian cuisine. Much later in life, I discovered its capacity to heal because of its powerful anti-inflammatory properties. Curcumin is the star medicinal compound in turmeric, and it has been shown to be effective in helping to treat conditions such as certain cancers, arthritis, and neurodegenerative conditions. It is also an effective pain reliever, rivaling over-the-counter medicines.

And for menopause? The benefits just keep coming. Recent studies have also indicated that curcumin:

Helps relieve hot flashes. One study, published in *Complementary Therapies in Medicine* in 2020, found that curcumin (200mg capsule daily) helped to reduce hot flashes.[7] Adding this spice to your diet might reduce the frequency and severity of your hot flashes if that's something you struggle with and wish to address.

Boost testosterone. By increasing testosterone levels, curcumin is thought to help increase sex drive in women.

Trim your physique. An analysis of multiple studies showed that curcumin intake was linked to reduced weight and waist circumference in sixteen hundred people.[8] This may be attributed to curcumin's inflammation-reducing properties.

Improve gut health. Curcumin has strong clinical evidence for treating gut health, including nausea, diarrhea, constipation, and more. With a healthy gut, many other menopause symptoms improve–I wrote a whole chapter on this. Improved gut health through the consumption of turmeric is all due to curcumin's antioxidant and anti-inflammatory properties. What's more, it's currently being studied as a potential treatment for irritable bowel syndrome, Crohn's disease, and ulcerative colitis.

Sharpen memory. With menopause comes brain fog, which affects memory. One clinical trial showed that curcumin improved memory in adults who did not have dementia. This could be attributed to its ability to lower inflammation in the brain.

Boost mood. Mood changes, depression, and anxiety are common in menopausal women and have detrimental impacts that proliferate in every aspect of life. Specifically, curcumin may be able to increase levels of chemicals in the brain that help combat depression, making it somewhat of a natural happy pill. Plus, it's delicious.

It's easy to obtain all these benefits by simply adding turmeric to various foods such as oatmeal, homemade sauces or dressings, curries, smoothies, green juices, rice, stews, soups, scrambled eggs, muffins, and many other foods. If you add a pinch of pepper along with turmeric, all the better. Pepper significantly boosts the availability–up to 2,000 percent.

Bone Density Loss

Estrogen also protects your bones by promoting the activity of *osteoblasts*, which are the cells that manufacture new bone. When estrogen levels drop—for example, during perimenopause—you may lose bone density, or the amount of minerals in your bone. The loss of bone density can increase the risk of fractures. As you progress through this transition, loss of bone-protecting estrogen may also put you at risk for osteoporosis, a serious condition characterized by weak and brittle bones. A bone density test can reveal the health and integrity of your bones. In general, though, women across the board experience dramatic drops in estrogen and vitamin D during perimenopause, meaning that most women are at higher risk of osteoporosis anyway due to these deficiencies. It is crucial that women are aware of this fact and can take steps to prevent bone loss.

Thinning Hair and Brittle Nails

Similar to what some women may experience during pregnancy, during perimenopause and menopause, hormonal fluctuations can impact hair follicles. As a result, your hair gets thinner and more brittle, and the texture of your hair can change as you age. These changes are mostly due to a decline in estrogen levels. More than half of women over age 50 deal with hair loss, according to recent research.[9]

Estrogen is the number one factor here, too. It has vasodilatory effects, meaning it helps dilate blood vessels and improve blood flow so that hair follicles get oxygen and nutrients. As estrogen tapers off, hair follicles are deprived of vital nutrients such as beta-carotene and omega-3 fats that help them thrive. For hair follicles to actively grow, they need large amounts of energy (calories). Producing a single gram of hair requires around thirty-eight calories of energy—so radical, starvation-type diets will not help you if your hair is thinning!

Not all women will have hair problems during the transition since the severity of changes can vary widely from woman to woman. Although the primary culprit behind hair loss during menopause is typically hormonal changes, there are many other factors (genetics, stress, diet, specific nutritional deficiencies, underlying health conditions, and the use of certain medications) that can affect hair health. Investigators have also now demonstrated that changes to our gut microbiome are linked to stress-related hair loss. Lots of women I work with complain of thinning hair, but after they change their diet and lifestyle, menopausal hair loss can be stopped and hair growth restored. There are so many hair-growth products out there marketed toward women, but as with all trendy products, it's important to read the labels for harmful ingredients and speak with your doctor before incorporating it into your routine.

In a similar vein, as estrogen levels fall off, so does the production of collagen and keratin—two proteins involved in the structure of nails, hair, and skin. Nail layers in particular weaken and become brittle.

Bloating

With a poor diet of processed foods, additives, and preservatives, your gut can't catch a break, and it becomes inflamed, even more so during perimenopause and menopause. Your gut bacteria aren't as balanced as they should be, the system breaks down, you can't properly digest food, and a host of problems sets in, one of which is bloating.

Compounding this problem are your erratic hormones. This causes water retention, which in turn leads to further bloating. Lifestyle factors such as diet and stress levels during menopause can also cause bloating related to excess gas. Luckily for you, there are tons of ways to minimize bloating through effective nutrition, exercise, and other lifestyle factors.

As for other digestive issues, hormones such as, you guessed it, estrogen affect your microbiome, the community of microorganisms living in your gut. When hormone levels start to fluctuate during perimenopause, the makeup of your microbiome may change, which can affect digestion. An unbalanced microbiome that leads to altered estrogen levels could have longer-term health implications. Adding to the misery is that an unbalanced microbiome leads to an increase in fat, changes in mood, and issues with sleep. Your gut bacteria can affect how different foods are digested and impact whether you feel full or not, which leads to overeating. The gut microbiome is powerful, and it's rarely if ever discussed pertaining to women's health and the hormonal continuum, which is why it's such a large portion of this book.

Itchy Skin

For tight, soft, and dewy skin, we need estrogen. It is involved in the production of collagen, the most abundant protein in the body. It keeps your skin moist and supple. We already know that when estrogen levels begin dropping off during perimenopause, so does collagen. This reduction leads to loss of skin elasticity and, with it, sagging and dry, itchy skin.

You might also develop chronic hives, characterized by mosquito-bite-type rashes on your skin. These are generally not allergic reactions, but due to hormonal changes that will resolve in time and with holistic treatment.

Dizziness

Here's a symptom you don't hear much about, but it is fairly common. Roller-coaster hormone levels that begin in perimenopause can mess with your inner ear and blood sugar levels in ways that may make you feel dizzy. And if you're feeling fatigued? Indirectly, fatigue during perimenopause can also cause you to feel dizzy. So can dehydration if night sweats and hot flashes are leaving you thirsty.

Heart Palpitations

Don't freak out if you feel a sudden, fast, panicky pounding in your chest. This menopausal symptom is quite common and caused by hormone fluctuations (isn't just about everything?). My mother started having erratic heartbeats during menopause, and it was quite scary at first. She had an entire cardiac workup, but further evaluation revealed the source of her problem was decreasing and sputtering hormones. Yes, this symptom is usually harmless, but if there are other symptoms like chest pain or dizziness along with it, please alert your health care provider.

Burning Mouth and Sense of Taste

Here's a fun fact: Your mouth contains receptors for sex hormones. As hormones bounce around during perimenopause, you might feel sensations of burning, numbness, and tingling on your tongue or in your mouth. Additionally, research estimates that up to 60 percent of women in this transition may experience some form of oral discomfort such as mouth or gum sensitivity and shifting teeth.[10] This same issue with sex hormone receptors in your mouth may also affect your sense of taste during perimenopause.

Allergies

Did you know that during perimenopause, you may experience new or worsening allergy symptoms? When your hormones fluctuate, histamine spikes, which causes itchiness. Histamine is a chemical that helps your body fight off invaders, but sometimes it overreacts and triggers allergies as part of your body's immune response.

Urinary Changes

Is your bladder misbehaving and you are not sure why? Several urinary changes during perimenopause are the culprit. One of the major ones is overactive bladder (OAB), characterized by a frequent or sudden urge to urinate. Another is urinary incontinence, meaning the involuntary loss of urine. It sometimes accompanies OAB.

What's more, perimenopause alters the balance of bacteria in your urogenital microbiome, the community of microorganisms that reside in your urinary and genital tracts. This change in the microbiome reduces the natural defense systems for fighting urinary tract infections, so you might be more susceptible to this problem. All these issues are related to changing hormone levels, which in turn lead to weakened muscles in your pelvic floor and changes in the lining of your bladder.

Tingling Limbs

A tingling sensation in the extremities isn't something we associate with menopause. However, hormone changes can affect your central nervous system (CNS) in such a way that some women periodically experience tingling in the hands, feet, arms, or legs for a few minutes at a time. Also starting during perimenopause, some women may experience sensations similar to an electric shock beneath the skin. These shocks likely occur because the electric impulses used as a signaling mechanism in the body to the brain are disrupted by hormone fluctuations during menopause. As mentioned earlier, estrogen is a neuroprotective hormone, whose decline may instigate shock-like sensations and related symptoms.

Body Odor

Several symptoms of menopause like hot flashes and night sweats can cause women to perspire more, which can then lead to changes in body odor. An increase in testosterone relative to the amount of estrogen in the body can also bump up the number of odor-causing bacteria present in sweat during menopause. Similarly, it's not uncommon to experience the onset of vaginal odor during menopause. This has to do with shifts experienced in the vaginal microbiome, which are commonly affected by fluctuations of hormone levels.

While these changes in body odor seem to pop up out of nowhere and can be frustrating, it's entirely normal and you are not alone. What worked for you in your twenties may not be what is best for your perimenopause body, and a new hygiene routine could be necessary to address changes in body odor associated with hormonal shifts. It may be tempting to purchase perfumed products that claim to make your body odor disappear, both for your armpits and lady bits. However, I strongly caution against using scented products on areas where the skin is sensitive, such as the vaginal area. Scented products, whether that be lotions, scented tampons, vaginal washes, exfoliating scrubs, and more contain chemicals that will alter pH, which can lead to irritation of the skin and even an infection.

Instead, make sure you are bathing frequently, especially after exercise, night sweats, or hot flashes if you can. You can continue to use scented lotions, deodorants, and perfumes as long as they don't cause irritation to the skin. Installing a bidet, which has become increasingly more affordable and widespread, is a good way to ensure hygiene down there throughout the day, thus minimizing vaginal odor. Finally, stay hydrated and make sure your diet isn't furthering the issue of increased body odor. Certain foods, especially when paired with high stress levels, can make body odor worse, independent of hormonal changes.

MENTAL CHANGES OF PERIMENOPAUSE

The laundry list of physical symptoms a woman can experience because of hormonal changes during perimenopause is astounding and, frankly, daunting. Through puberty, adulthood, pregnancy, perimenopause, and beyond, the female hormonal continuum is fraught with drastic, often uncontrollable changes to the body that can be difficult to manage or cope with. Every woman experiences her hormonal continuum differently, and unfortunately there are too few treatment options for women experiencing unruly side effects; we're just expected to endure life in the midst of pain from our cycle or deal with annoying perimenopause symptoms on our own. When I entered this stage of life, I knew I needed to offer some much-needed help to readers—we don't have to suffer in silence anymore!

Beyond the physical symptoms of perimenopause and menopause, many women face significant psychological changes that can have a tremendous impact on not only our mental health but also our physical health, worsening the already bothersome physical side effects of hormonal transition. Women in perimenopause are more at risk of mood disturbances, relapse or worsening of preexisting mental disorders, and increased anxiety than women pre- or postmenopause. The following is a list of mental symptoms you may experience during perimenopause. It may be surprising, perhaps overwhelming, to see every symptom laid out in this way, but it's important to bring awareness to these often unseen side effects of progressing along the hormonal continuum. This part of the experience will often be the hurdle that tests us the most. The mind can trick us into fear and stagnancy, but I encourage you to work against those odds, using the tools outlined in this book.

Mood Changes

Starting during perimenopause, don't be surprised if you get more moody than usual. Around one in five women may deal with mood swings during perimenopause through postmenopause, and they are bothersome. Brought on by hormone fluctuations, you may experience mood swings as well as increased feelings of anger, sadness, stress, or irritability. Changes in mood can intensify toward the end of perimenopause.

You might be surprised to find yourself easily angered and frustrated over the least little things, often without even realizing it. This can cause strain on relationships in your life, and it's easy to blame yourself for outbursts you can't explain. For context, your increased irritability may be related to hormone fluctuations but compounded by other perimenopause issues like poor sleep and stress. Rather than get upset at yourself for feeling like your emotions are out of control, try to think of ways to address them, like journaling, having alone time to decompress, enjoying a hobby or exercise, or through your diet.

Quick Pause: Irritable Today? Have These Foods on Hand

When your estrogen levels dip, so does the neurotransmitter serotonin, produced mostly in the gut and responsible for keeping our moods on an even keel. Serotonin (also known as the happiness hormone) is derived from tryptophan (an amino acid in food). If you find yourself feeling depressed, experiencing insomnia, or having low self-esteem during the menopause transition, odds are you may need a serotonin boost–and you can do that by choosing some specific foods.

For example: Eat foods high in tryptophan, including eggs, turkey, dairy, lean meats, salmon, pineapple, tofu, nuts, and seeds–but mix them with quality carbohydrates such as sweet potatoes, winter squashes, and quinoa. In fact, I advise that if you add meat or other animal proteins to your diet, they should account for only about 10 percent of the food on your plate.

Carbohydrates are important because they help drive tryptophan across the blood-brain barrier (BBB), a protective membrane that covers the brain. The BBB prevents toxins from reaching the brain, while allowing vital nutrients to enter.

Enjoy foods high in vitamin B₆, which is also important for serotonin production. Vitamin B₆ is plentiful in cauliflower, bananas, avocado, grains, nuts, and seeds.

Other mood-lifting foods during the menopause transition include those high in vitamin D and omega-3 fatty acids, says a study published in 2023 in the journal *Menopause*.[11] Vitamin D-rich foods include fatty fish (think salmon, tuna, and mackerel), mushrooms, and egg yolks. For a burst of omega-3 fats, too, reach for fatty fish, oysters, flaxseeds, chia seeds, walnuts, and soybeans.

Depression

The hormonal swings that begin during perimenopause may make you more prone to depression, especially if you've dealt with depression in the past, but other factors may be involved. These include weight gain, problems related to your sex life, and life changes (think divorce, loss of a parent, children leaving home, sick relatives, and so forth). Women who have never struggled with depression are also at risk of experiencing first-onset depression during perimenopause due to a variety of factors, including the physical symptoms they experience during hormonal transition. A recent study found that women who do not struggle with perimenopausal symptoms are less likely to be diagnosed with a psychiatric disorder during this stage of the hormonal continuum.[12] If you think you may be exhibiting signs of depression, regardless if you've ever received a prior diagnosis, I encourage you to seek professional help from your primary care doctor or a therapist to discuss a treatment plan, whether that be medication, cognitive therapy, or other means. Your feelings are valid, your symptoms are valid, and you don't have to endure this journey alone.

Anxiety

Again, fluctuating hormones, along with sleep disturbances and other lifestyle changes, can all provoke anxiety during perimenopause. By anxiety, I'm referring to feelings of nervousness or impending danger, increased heart rate (including palpitations), sweating, trouble sleeping, digestive problems, and a feeling of general unrest. Women who suffer from physical symptoms of perimenopause are more likely to experience increased anxiety, as they do with depression. The intense and ongoing anxiety we feel manifests in the form of physiological stress, which can take a toll on our sleep, energy levels, mood, digestion, posture, and aspects of our social and professional lives. Luckily, there are tons of ways to modify your lifestyle to minimize anxiety, which we'll go over in later chapters.

Panic Disorder

In some women, declining estrogen and progesterone during the menopausal transition can trigger unexpected and unexplained panic attacks. These are sudden episodes of intense anxiety in which you feel a sense of impending doom and experience alarming physical symptoms, such as a racing heartbeat, shortness of breath, or nausea. For women struggling with panic attacks, speaking with a licensed professional may provide much needed support, as might medication on an as-needed basis.

Brain Fog and Memory Problems

Having trouble concentrating? You are definitely not alone here, either. Experts say that about 66 percent of women report having difficulty taking in and remembering new information during this transition—a problem commonly referred to as "brain fog."[13] I struggled with brain fog for a long time, not understanding why it felt like I couldn't think clearly, like I wasn't at my best and wouldn't ever be again. However, I dug into research and discovered that brain fog is a widespread symptom of perimenopause—there were other women out there going through the same thing as I was, yet I had never heard anyone discuss it and how hard it was to get through the day sometimes. Why?

Well, changing hormone levels are mostly to blame. The decline in estrogen that begins during perimenopause can lead to feelings of mental fogginess—as can poor sleep caused by night sweats or another one of the thirty-four symptoms of menopause, such as stress and anxiety.

For the female brain, estrogen is a neuroprotective hormone that guards your brain, nerves, and their functions from damage. It keeps brain cells healthy and active and fosters normal activity in regions associated with memory, concentration, and organization. Estrogen also helps forge new connections among brain cells, which makes the brain more resilient and adaptable. Because we need estrogen for brain health, it's easy to see why declines in estrogen in the brain can lead to brain fog, increased likelihood of dementia, and possibly other brain problems.

Like brain fog, memory problems during the menopausal transition are often linked to changing hormone levels. About 62 percent of women in perimenopause and menopause report declines in cognitive performance, including memory.[14] With my protocol, you'll learn a lot about how to protect your brain health throughout the hormonal continuum.

ARE THERE OTHER SYMPTOMS THAT MIGHT SET OFF ALARMS?

Definitely. There are some perimenopause symptoms that are not normal. For example, one of the most worrisome symptoms is abnormal bleeding, which could point to underlying problems with your reproductive system or organs. Get in touch with your physician or OB-GYN right away if you're experiencing any of the following:

- Bleeding so heavily that you need to change your tampons or pads every hour or two. This can be a sign of fibroids, infection, a sexually transmitted disease, a thyroid problem, endometrial polyps, or, in very rare cases, cancer.
- Bleeding that continues for longer than 7 days.
- "Breakthrough bleeding," which occurs between periods.
- Periods that regularly occur less than 21 days apart.
- Bleeding during or after sex.

TRACK YOUR SYMPTOMS

Knowing where you are with your symptoms is key to addressing them. Ask yourself: What are my symptoms? How severe are they? How often do they occur?

To help you, I've put together this symptom tracker. It will make you more aware of what's going on and help you have an open discussion with your health care provider about the changes taking place in your body.

Instructions: Circle "Yes" if you're currently experiencing or have experienced the listed symptom recently. Then describe the duration, frequency, and severity in the corresponding text box. Circle "No" if you're not experiencing the listed symptom. Use this checklist, along with your lab results (FSH, TSH, vitamin D, and so on) to work with your primary care physician or OB-GYN.

Knowing where you are *now* will point you in the direction of becoming the healthy woman you know you can be. I wrote this book as a resource for anyone whose symptoms were not taken seriously or for anyone who has ever asked themselves, "Is this normal?"

Symptoms	Circle	If "YES," describe duration (how long does it last?), frequency (how often does it occur?), and severity (on a scale from 1 to 5, with 5 being the most severe)
Hot flashes	Yes or No	
Night sweats	Yes or No	
Irregular periods	Yes or No	
Weight changes	Yes or No	
Breast tenderness	Yes or No	
Sleep issues	Yes or No	

Fatigue	Yes or No	
Vaginal dryness	Yes or No	
Lower sex drive	Yes or No	
Headaches	Yes or No	
Joint pain	Yes or No	
Muscle aches	Yes or No	
Bone loss	Yes or No	
Thinning hair	Yes or No	
Brittle nails	Yes or No	
Bloating	Yes or No	
Other digestive issues	Yes or No	
Itchy skin	Yes or No	
Dizziness	Yes or No	
Heart palpitations	Yes or No	
Burning tongue and/or mouth	Yes or No	
Altered sense of taste	Yes or No	
Allergies	Yes or No	
Urinary changes	Yes or No	

Tingling limbs	Yes or No	
Body odor	Yes or No	
Mood changes	Yes or No	
Irritability	Yes or No	
Depression	Yes or No	
Anxiety	Yes or No	
Panic disorder	Yes or No	
Brain fog	Yes or No	
Memory problems	Yes or No	

I know this chapter is overwhelming—everything about being a woman, having hormones that are constantly changing, aging, and juggling the responsibilities of life, is overwhelming. My hope is that as you've read through the various symptoms, physical and mental, of perimenopause, you're able to put your finger on exactly what you've been feeling. Trouble sleeping, weight gain, fluctuating mood? You aren't crazy; you might just be in perimenopause. As a medical professional, I hope to demystify the vast world of women's health and both validate the experience of women everywhere and provide them with information and tools to take charge of their health.

CHAPTER 3

Hormone Therapy and Other FAQs

D R. SHAH, AM I IN perimenopause?"
"Does this apply to me?"
"What about hormone therapy?"
"Can I still get pregnant?"
"How do I know when I'll be in menopause?"

These are just some of the questions I get on a regular basis. Most of you are reading this book because you're in perimenopause or menopause right now or you think you might be. By now, you've probably identified certain symptoms that you may experience on a regular basis, but I'm sure there are still a ton of questions floating around in your mind. In this chapter I'll do my best to answer your burning questions related to all things hormone therapy and the body during perimenopause and menopause.

We still have a long way to go to fully understand the physiological and hormonal changes during perimenopause and menopause, especially since every woman experiences them in her own way, depending on her health and other factors. Perimenopause is perhaps the grayest area on the hormonal continuum in that most of us don't even notice we've progressed into this stage until we are well into the transition. I've heard from many women that they didn't realize perimenopause was a term to describe what comes before the big M, menopause. You don't go from being fertile to menopausal in a day, and I'm here to help you navigate the in-between. Whether your goals are to fix your gut microbiome, try for an advanced maternal–aged pregnancy, minimize your hormone-related symptoms, strengthen your body, improve your relationship with food, or prolong your life, the tools I've provided you in this book can help you get there.

My best advice for women who aren't sure where they are on the hormonal continuum is to keep a diary to catalog your cycles, symptoms, and how you feel. You can use the chart at the end of the previous chapter, or you can create one on your own, personalized to your unique journey. Maybe you notice that your quality of sleep has significantly diminished in the past year and you're experiencing hot flashes and irritability more frequently. Maybe your cycles have become more irregular. Maybe your libido isn't what it was a year ago. When these details are tracked consistently over a prolonged period of time, you will begin to notice variations across the years, months, and even weeks that will give you a more defined portrait of your hormonal transition.

Once you've determined that you're in perimenopause and you want to manage the symptoms you identified through your diary, start keeping track of your nutrition (not your calories), exercise, and sleep. We'll talk more about this in Part II, but it's worth mentioning now to get you thinking about your lifestyle habits and how they may be working with or against your hormones. The best way to improve your gut health is through knowing what is going on in your body, how you are feeling, and how you are fueling your body and mind. When you make changes in your diet and lifestyle centered on improving your gut health, you will notice that these other areas of your health will improve as well.

As you may recall, menopause is the point at which your ovaries stop functioning and you have 12 consecutive months without a period. Women can experience symptoms of menopause from 4 to up to 14 years. Even today, researchers don't fully understand the reason behind this tremendous gap in how women experience menopause.

If you're over the age of 35, prioritizing exercise and nutrition isn't just about "looking good" anymore. It's about preserving your brain volume, muscle mass, and bone density, all of which can decline by 3 to 5 percent every decade after age 30. I don't know about you, but my goal is to grow into the strong, fierce old lady that I know

I can be postmenopause. For now, though, I still have menopause to contend with.

HORMONE THERAPY

There's a lot of talk about hormone therapy online, and I suspect that many of you picked up this book partially because you're looking for answers on whether it may be right for you. The short answer? Well, maybe.

To get a handle on their hormones and manage menopausal symptoms, many women turn to menopausal hormone therapy (MHT), sometimes referred to as hormone replacement therapy (HRT). MHT and HRT are sometimes used interchangeably, but the main difference is that HRT refers to treatment for conditions outside of menopause and often for people younger than 40. MHT is the more appropriate term to use when describing supplemental hormone treatment specifically for symptoms of menopause. If you've been saying "HRT" when referring to MHT, that's okay! I'm not here to be the grammar police—I just want you to be aware of the distinction and equip you with the knowledge to make smart health decisions and hopefully spot misinformation floating around on social media.

The topic of hormone therapy has been the subject of hot debate for decades, and many women, even doctors, feel conflicted about its place in managing menopause symptoms. For a long time, hormone therapy was a popular option for treating menopause-related symptoms before it fell out of fashion due to potential links to cancer and other serious side effects in the early 2000s.[1] Since then, claims that hormone therapy is dangerous have been seriously refuted, and it has slowly crept back into the mainstream conversations surrounding menopause. However, as of 2023, 1.8 percent of menopausal women are using some form of hormone therapy, down from 4.6 percent in 2007, despite its resurgence in discussions within online spaces.[2] Note that this statistic from The Menopause Society is talking only about women in menopause, and it does not reflect the percentage of postmenopausal women who are on hormone therapy—I suspect that number exceeds 1.8 percent, but this data has not been collected. Regardless, this indicates to me that women are curious about hormone therapy, but they may be hesitant to pursue it. It's only natural that you have questions about hormone therapy as an option for your symptoms, and this chapter is solely dedicated to unraveling the complicated and often misunderstood reality of hormone therapy.

TYPES AND PURPOSES OF MHT

Beyond the distinction between HRT and MHT, there are different types of hormone therapies a doctor may prescribe to a patient struggling with menopause symptoms. The first type is known as *systemic therapy*, wherein hormones such as estrogens and progestogens (like progesterone) are administered in the form of pills, a vaginal ring, or topical sprays, gels, or patches. The route of administration (ROA) and form of systemic therapy you may be prescribed will vary depending on your provider's availability of resources, your medical coverage, and of course your medical history and doctor's guidance. In the same way that different forms of birth control can have vastly different side effects on a patient, so, too, can MHT. Hormones delivered through systemic therapy are absorbed into the bloodstream at a high rate, making it a popular course of treatment for hot flashes, for example. It's also used to protect bone health in patients with low bone density, or osteoporosis.

The second type is *low-dose therapy*, sometimes referred to as *vaginal estrogen therapy*. Hormones are administered into the vagina to help replenish tissues and moisture within the vaginal canal. Low-dose therapy hormones are not absorbed into the bloodstream at a high rate as with systemic therapy, so the overall risks and side effects (I'll discuss this in more depth a bit later in this section) of this type of MHT are much lower.

Within these two types of MHT, your doctor may prescribe you estrogen-only variations of MHT, or a combination of estrogen and progesterone, EPT. Generally, if you've had a hysterectomy that means you no longer need progesterone and will benefit most from estrogen-only MHT. For those who still have a uterus, EPT will be the most effective form of MHT in its role of preventing endometrial cancer as opposed to estrogen-only therapy, which thickens the uterine lining and increases the risk of this type of cancer. Estrogen-only MHT and EPT have different ROAs and dose frequency, so they are not interchangeable—these are things you should ask your doctor about when considering hormone therapy for menopause symptoms.

Quick Pause: What Are "Bioidentical Hormones"?

If you're a middle-aged woman on social media, you've likely seen ads for hormone clinics, menopause products, hormone pellets, and these things called "bioidentical hormones." This term is a strategic way for wellness companies to make you think it's better and more natural than traditional MHT, but that's just not true. "Bioidentical" is a marketing term. Let me explain.

First things first: Hormones used for traditional MHT are often "bioidentical" in that they can have the same chemical makeup as the hormones produced naturally in the body. Some FDA-approved hormones prescribed by medical doctors and used in traditional MHT fit under this definition of "bioidentical," even if they aren't talked about or marketed in that way. There are also synthetic hormones (not chemically identical) that are FDA approved, used in traditional MHT, and designed to have the same biological effects as our naturally occurring hormones. Bioidentical and synthetic hormones are both created in a lab, typically derived from plants, and what matters isn't so much how identical they are to your hormones or how "natural" they may seem but rather how they affect the body.

The term *bioidentical hormones* is used to promote something that's more accurately described as "custom-compounded hormones," which are not approved nor regulated by the FDA and are not proven to be better or more effective than traditional forms of MHT. While the hormones used for some bioidentical (read: "custom-compounded") therapies may be the same as ones used for traditional MHT (like estrone, estradiol, DHEA, progesterone, or testosterone), the reality of this customization process results in too many unknown variables such as incorrect dosage, poor quality, and the fact that they are not tested for safety or absorption into the bloodstream. Companies market their products as tailored to the patient's needs, but that isn't something exclusive to alternative hormone therapies. When doctors prescribe traditional MHT and synthetic hormones, they are taking into account the patient's symptoms and health history, and monitoring the patient's response to MHT to assess the efficacy of the dosage and the ROA.

Bioidentical hormone therapy can be administered via pill, patch, gel, cream, or injection. A popular form of bioidentical hormone therapy is administered in the form of a pellet, around the size of a grain of rice, under the skin. A pharmacy will custom-compound the bioidentical hormone pellet according to a prescription from a doctor, and then a medical professional will implant the pellet under the skin. Some view it as a safer alternative to traditional MHT, but there is not yet sufficient evidence to support this opinion. Further, most hormone experts do not recommend pellet therapy because it's not easy to monitor and people could be getting much higher doses than what they need. If dosed incorrectly and over an extended period of time, a patient's risk of certain cancers, blood clots, and other issues could be greatly increased. I do think there could be safe options for compounded bioidentical hormone therapy out there depending on the pharmacy, but at the moment we don't have a regulating body looking at these products, guaranteeing their safety, and ruling out the good from the bad. It is my hope that more research is done on bioidentical custom-compounded hormone therapy and the FDA can regulate these products; there's so much potential for this method to help women in menopause, but it's an area that needs further study.

In my professional opinion, I don't recommend bioidentical pellet therapy simply because there are so many things we don't know about it in terms of safety, both short-term and long-term, and its effectiveness as compared to proven methods of traditional MHT. However, if you do decide to go with bioidentical pellet therapy, only do so because you are with a trusted pharmacy and you have discussed it with your doctor. For most people I know, once they understand how MHT works and the different types and risks, they choose to stick with traditional forms of MHT rather than seek riskier alternative options.

Negative side effects of MHT can include nausea, irregular bleeding, spotting, changes in mood, breast tenderness, skin irritation, and headaches. These side effects are common, though not everyone on MHT will experience them. It may also be difficult for people using MHT to distinguish these symptoms from menopause symptoms in that they can be very similar. Apart from annoying side effects, some known (though uncommon and extreme) risks associated with MHT include blood clots, uterine cancer (for those who still have their uterus), breast cancer, and even a small risk of stroke. Women who have taken MHT have a 24 percent greater risk of breast cancer than women who have never taken MHT.[3] While both estrogen-only and EPT forms of MHT are associated with an increased risk of breast cancer, women taking EPT have an even greater risk of breast cancer for reasons we are still trying to understand. In particular, women on MHT have an increased likelihood of developing a slow-progressing form of breast cancer called luminal A; this subtype of breast cancer makes up over 60 percent of breast cancer cases and has a good prognosis. Breast cancer survivors may be discouraged from EPT due to an elevated risk of reoccurrence of cancerous tumors. Regardless, these risks increase over time the longer you are treated with MHT. Beginning MHT within ten years of your last cycle is generally considered safe practice, but starting it outside of that window increases risk for developing breast cancer, heart disease, blood clots, and even stroke. Per The Menopause Society, it is recommended that women treated with MHT stop after four to five years, gradually lowering their dose to help minimize the risk of adverse effects as well as the chances of symptoms such as hot flashes returning.[4]

While the risks MHT poses are serious and can be life-threatening in extreme cases, there are many known benefits of MHT and its effectiveness in addressing some of the more uncomfortable menopause symptoms. MHT can decrease the severity and frequency of hot flashes, night sweats, changes in mood, and help with vaginal dryness as well as sleep and brain fog. As stated before, MHT can help protect your bones, and it can ease symptoms of an overactive bladder. It may also reduce your risk of developing cardiovascular disease and type 2 diabetes. You can rest assured that MHT does not *cause* breast cancer as many used to believe, yet every person considering MHT should carefully weigh the risks before starting treatment.

IS MHT RIGHT FOR ME?

I'll give you my opinion, but remember that this is a conversation that should be had with your doctor if you're curious about how hormone therapy might help you. Not everyone going through perimenopause or menopause needs to be on hormone therapy. In fact, there are only three specific factors that indicate when a person might benefit from hormone therapy.

The three main indicators for being a strong candidate for MHT are:

1. You're having hot flashes and night sweats.
2. You currently have or are at high risk of osteoporosis.
3. You're experiencing vaginal dryness or discomfort.

I was talking to my OB-GYN bestie (she's an MHT specialist) after yoga one morning and asked her, "How do you make a decision for people like me in their forties, who have periods, but are not sure about signs of perimenopause after fixing their gut health?"

Before correcting my diet, I struggled with a ton of symptoms that I thought could be early perimenopause. But after I improved my diet and sleep, most of these symptoms lessened or disappeared entirely. While I was thrilled to be feeling better in my body, I felt more confused than ever about my place on the hormonal continuum.

My bestie is in a similar situation, and we're close in age; it was so validating to talk to an expert who can also closely relate to what I'm personally going through. We spent a while discussing whether we would be good candidates for MHT. It's trending (once again) for brain, heart, muscle, and skin benefits, and women are treating it like a fountain of youth. I'll admit, all the buzz got me wondering, "Is this something I need to be considering in my life right now?" It's highly subjective. Long story short, neither me nor my bestie currently experience the big three symptoms, and we both decided to wait on pursuing MHT until we feel that our symptoms are out of the normal level of discomfort, meaning they are disruptive to sleep and other aspects of health. I can't express how valuable it is to have a partner in perimenopause (PIP); we maintain an open dialogue about how we're feeling and agreed to reassess our symptoms with each other every three months as a way to hold ourselves accountable and keep our health in check.

This is a highly nuanced discussion that should be had with your doctor based on symptoms and risk. However, I encourage you to find a PIP of your own, someone close in age who may be experiencing similar things as you. If we allow ourselves to be open with others about what we're feeling, it's a lot easier to identify when we should seek out a doctor's guidance and treatment. If I started MHT tomorrow, the benefits at this point in my journey on the hormonal continuum would be unclear since my symptoms aren't intense. It's still a medication, after all, and I don't want to be introducing new medications to my body unless it's something I truly need. I'm not saying a strong no to MHT forever, but right now it isn't a necessity for me, and it certainly is not for everyone.

If you don't struggle with the big 3 symptoms, hormone therapy may be an unnecessary measure in helping you navigate hormonal transition. For those of you who do suffer from one or all these big indicators, hormone therapy could be a good option to consider, but be advised that hormone therapy alone will not magically fix your symptoms. With or without MHT, you will still advance through perimenopause and menopause, and your body will go through significant changes. Starting MHT during perimenopause to subvert some of the more extreme symptoms of menopause could pose unnecessary risks to a variety of aspects of your health. MHT *does not* allow you to escape the inevitable.

I've noticed some discourse online treating MHT as a sort of antiaging potion. Sorry to burst your bubble, but that's just simply not the case. It doesn't restore youth. People think it'll be a shortcut to feeling and looking good. If anything, the surge in MHT's recent popularity has further intensified the stigma about aging. Let me be very clear: MHT is not good or evil. It is purely a medical treatment to alleviate discomfort from hormone-related symptoms. While I am critical of some of the ways MHT is discussed online, I am also incredibly grateful for my colleagues out there spreading awareness about MHT as a viable option for treatment. The more women are educated on aspects of women's health beyond puberty and pregnancy, the less women will suffer as they progress along the continuum. Increased education about perimenopause, menopause, and MHT will without a doubt result in decreased suffering across the board.

NOT *EITHER-OR* BUT *AND*

I recently had a 56-year-old patient, let's call her Lupita, who came to me about her menopause symptoms. She has a rare blood-clotting disorder, which makes her unable to be on MHT as it could put her at further risk of life-threatening blood clots. Lupita expressed her concerns about some of her menopause symptoms such as hair thinning, skin dryness, poor sleep, and her worries of one day having dementia. She had heard that many women use MHT to combat these issues, and she felt distress over not being able to take MHT, thinking it was the only way to manage menopause symptoms and prevent dementia. These are valid worries, and many women out there are in similar situations.

Rest assured that MHT is not the only way to address menopause symptoms. A lot of people think it will help them lose weight, clear their brain fog, or help them sleep better, but for a lot of women, that isn't their experience with MHT at all. While MHT is great for helping specific symptoms, it isn't going to be a cure-all for every symptom or every woman. I spoke with Lupita about various things she could change in her lifestyle to get the results she wanted, such as cutting alcohol and taking more walks in nature to protect her brain health, following the 30–30–3 (see chapter 4) to improve her gut health, and better sleep hygiene as well as nonhormonal options for addressing hot flashes.

Lupita left our appointment feeling reassured that being ineligible for MHT was not the end of the world. She walked away with a plan based on our conversation, and she was excited to implement these small changes that could benefit her in ways she thought only MHT could.

I thought I'd share this patient story to help paint a more nuanced picture of the MHT conversation with hopes that some readers can see themselves in Lupita. If you aren't a good candidate for MHT, there are so many other ways you can treat your menopause symptoms.

When thinking about strategies for managing your symptoms, don't approach this from an "either-or" standpoint but rather from a place of "and." Let me explain.

This entire book is about the intersection of nutrition and the hormonal continuum; when your gut health improves, all areas of the body, including your hormones, will benefit from having a stronger, more diverse gut microbiome. Starting hormone therapy for osteoporosis, for example, may serve to reverse the loss of bone density, but it will not address other deficiencies in the way that eating a nutrient-rich diet will. Whether or not hormone therapy is right for you, everyone should be following the 30–30–3, getting adequate sleep and exercise, and taking care of their body.

Here's another patient story: A 54-year-old patient, let's call her

Annie, began taking MHT in her early forties, yet she was struggling with fatigue, hair loss, and weight gain. She was wondering why she was still experiencing these symptoms despite being on MHT and what she could do about it. I explained that MHT alone won't be enough to see the changes she wanted and that we should look to her diet and lifestyle. I recommended she follow the 30–30–3 with special focus on getting more protein. We set a goal for her to take more walks outside, and with a weighted vest when possible, to promote a healthier morning routine centered around physical activity and mindfulness. After 3 months, Annie came back to me feeling like a different person. Her menopause symptoms decreased, and she felt better than she had when she was just taking MHT to treat her symptoms.

Hormone therapy is not a quick fix for menopause, though it can help many people manage some of the more debilitating symptoms. For the record, I have menopausal and postmenopausal patients who are currently on MHT and thriving; I also have patients at these same stages of life who are thriving without MHT. Regardless of whether a patient is or isn't on MHT, the point I'm trying to get across is that your health can be optimized first through nutrition. Maybe you and your doctor decide that hormone therapy is right for you. That's great! Don't lose focus on your diet, exercise, and sleep, though. MHT alone will not help you optimize the mind-gut connection, but MHT *and* positive lifestyle habits will. Taking an "either-or" approach to navigating menopause oversimplifies the many processes within the body. A comprehensive approach that consists of multiple complementary strategies for hormone health and longevity will give you the most benefits, even after menopause.

OTHER FREQUENTLY
ASKED QUESTIONS

How do I know if a symptom is related to my hormones and menopause or if it's something else?

How's your gut? Do you know your baseline? For example, is your sleep quality poor because you're drinking caffeine too late in the day? What's your sugar intake like? Are you getting enough whole foods in your diet? Once you curb unhelpful habits, you can achieve your so-called baseline to tell the hormone-related symptoms from the negative consequences of unhealthy lifestyle choices.

However, if your symptoms go deeper than poor sleep, gradual weight gain, or other common menopause symptoms, then schedule an appointment with your primary care doctor. Your doctor will be able to help you figure out what's going on, determine if something could be hormone-related, and recommend you see your OB-GYN or a different specialist. For example, if you notice you're gaining weight rapidly and you experience swelling of the limbs, there's a high likelihood those symptoms aren't just because you're approaching menopause and rather an indication of a serious underlying health condition.

I'll always advocate for lifestyle changes in lieu of introducing a new medication, but if changing diet and sleep are not improving a patient's symptoms, or if their symptoms are extreme and unusual, the next step is to run tests and work with them on getting to the root of the issue, whether that be hormone-related or a different and new undiagnosed medical condition. Many symptoms of other health conditions can mimic those of menopause, so when a doctor is presented with a woman in her fifties complaining of weight gain and night sweats, they are often too quick to write it off as simply the body's natural response to declining hormones and aging.

By the way, if you're someone whose doctor dismisses your concerns and writes off your symptoms as "being in your head" or "it's just your hormones," do not be afraid to get a second opinion. You know your body, and if it's telling you something is wrong, listen to it. Women literally die because of overconfident or inattentive doctors. As a doctor myself, I can acknowledge that none of us is perfect. I would rather a patient seek a second opinion (and potentially get life-saving care) than continue to suffer unnecessarily.

This is yet another reason why a symptom tracker is so incredibly important; beyond personal reference, the more accurate your documentation of what your body is doing, the better you can communicate what you're experiencing to get the treatment you need.

For example, if you've been having heart palpitations and bouts of dizziness that have steadily increased over the past 10 weeks, that's something your doctor should know. These are unusual menopause symptoms and could be an indicator that something else is causing these changes. A symptom tracker or journal is one of your best tools for advocating for your needs as a patient.

What if I think I might be going into menopause early?

It's possible! But not likely. Do you have regular periods, but you also have crazy hot flashes? You're not alone and not necessarily entering menopause anytime soon. Make sure you're tracking your cycles and symptoms, as this will help you gauge where you're at. If you still have regular periods but struggle with common menopause symptoms, this will typically mean you are solidly in the peri-menopause stage of the continuum. Remember, this can last a while, usually more than just a few years. If you're younger than 45, have irregular periods, and are experiencing common menopause symptoms, here are some steps to help you navigate the possibility of early menopause:

Step 1: Consider health factors that could cause you to enter menopause prematurely such as a family history of early menopause, a hysterectomy, certain autoimmune disorders, a history of medical treatments such as chemo or radiation, and even other factors like stress level and weight (particularly if you are underweight).

Step 2: Make an appointment with your OB-GYN to get your vitamin D tested and discuss the factors identified in step one. Your doctor will take it from here and work with you to determine a plan for care.

What will happen to my sex life?

Darling, your sex life can be whatever you want it to be before, during, and after menopause. But if you're curious about the bodily changes you will experience during menopause and how that will affect intimacy, I have some answers for you.

The first thing you need to know is that vaginal dryness is incredibly common the more your estrogen levels decrease, which can make intercourse painful. The weakening of the pelvic floor muscles after childbirth and through perimenopause exacerbates the issue.

Vaginal dryness and pain during sex are common reasons why some women seek MHT. However, if your libido is low, you no longer initiate sex, and you struggle with hypoactive sexual desire disorder (HSDD), you may also consider testosterone replacement therapy (TRT) under the guidance of your doctor. Most women will not require supplemental testosterone, and vaginal discomfort as well as low sex drive can instead be improved through other means such as vaginal moisturizers or lubricants, low-dose vaginal estrogen (a form of MHT), pelvic floor therapy, a healthy lifestyle, and even spicing things up in the bedroom now and then.

Many women may feel timid bringing up questions surrounding sex when talking about menopause, but these are valid concerns. The changes happening throughout the body during menopause can absolutely have an impact on what happens between the sheets (and I'm not just talking about night sweats). It can be daunting to face changes in your sex life amid the myriad other challenges a transition such as menopause already poses.

My nonmedical advice? Communicate with your partner. Be open about what you are going through and any discomfort you experience. It's important to keep an open line of communication here and set boundaries. If you feel that your hormone-related symptoms are taking a negative toll on your relationship with sex, I encourage you to consult your OB-GYN on paths for treatment, which could include MHT.

Can I still get pregnant if I'm in perimenopause?

Yes. In theory, if you are not on any form of birth control, still get a period, and have not had a hysterectomy, there's a possibility you could become pregnant during perimenopause.

Remember that your reserve of healthy eggs declines over the course of your life and that the eggs you retain after age 30 will decline in quality, leading to potential issues with fertility. Advanced maternal age (AMA), formerly known as geriatric pregnancy, refers to pregnancies that occur after the age of 35. These pregnancies are higher risk than pregnancies at younger ages, but it is still very common for women over 35 to have a typical pregnancy and deliver a healthy baby.

What you need to know is that getting pregnant over the age of 35 can mean an increased risk of miscarriage, gestational diabetes, stillbirth, fetal chromosomal abnormalities (such as Down syndrome), delivery via C-section, and other complications. If you want to try for pregnancy, but you think you might be in perimenopause, consult your OB-GYN for guidance given the natural decline in fertility and high-risk nature of these pregnancies.

Do I still need regular checkups and Pap smears with my OB-GYN?

Yes. Please, for all that you hold sacred, do not stop seeing an OB-GYN after you're done having children and/or if you've already gone through menopause. Just because you're postmenopausal does not mean your reproductive organs disappear and you're suddenly immune to threats like breast cancer, cervical cancer, and a long list of other issues.

Your yearly checkups, pelvic exams, and Pap smears are vital preventative care that are essential in catching cancer early. OB-GYNs also help patients with urinary incontinence, pelvic floor issues, sexual health, vaginal atrophy, and—you guessed it—prescribe MHT. Regular checkups with your OB-GYN also ensure up-to-date health data that your other providers can cross-reference to deliver effective care accurate to your needs. As if you needed another reason to keep your OB-GYN close, they are going to be your best ally in navigating life postmenopause. Your OB-GYN is there for you long after your last cycle.

CHAPTER 4

Gut Check

DURING MY TIME AS A medical student researching nutrition, I did a semester in the city. I was raptly interested in gut health–related foods, so I would frequently go to health food stores and get products marketed as high in fiber and good for your gut. Much to my dismay, a lot of these foods ended up containing high amounts of artificial sugars, harsh fibers, and alcohol sugars.

Like many people fooled by clever marketing, I was none the wiser and bought these products thinking they would help improve my gut health. I was sorely mistaken. After a few weeks, I was so bloated and had the worst abdominal pain of my life. I remember eating these snacks at the library and shortly after experiencing these cramps sent straight from hell. It was so bad that I had to lie down on the floor—in the library among my peers—to relieve the pain. That moment opened my eyes to how powerful the gut microbiome is, for better or worse. Our gut microbiome is complex, and processed food—even food that's marketed as healthy—can mess with your gut health.

Throughout the rest of this book, I'll be talking about perimenopause and health optimization strategies through the lens of the gut-brain axis. The intersection of women's health, hormones, and nutrition is rarely discussed, but that's where I come in. I'll teach you how to use food and supportive mind-gut strategies to your advantage during perimenopause and beyond to help you realize that your best years are not behind you.

Now, let's discover the wondrous world of the gut microbiome.

We know the gut is a highly complex part of the body, and it's important that you understand exactly what's going on in there. Bear with me as we dive into the inner workings of the gut microbiome, and I'll try my best to make this chapter as painless as possible. Your gut microbiome is an entire ecosystem unto itself, made up of trillions of microbes that can influence your appetite, mood, and health in a variety of ways, many of which we're just beginning to understand. I'll explain this in greater depth later in this chapter. But for now, imagine a commander in your gut with a walkie-talkie communicating to the commander in your brain about *everything*. The gut is like a command center speaking to another command center, the brain, to influence your hormones, immune system, and more. This is how important your gut is in your overall health.

"I was forty-five when I first started getting symptoms, and at first, I didn't realize what was happening," Sara told me at our appointment. "When I started noticing more bloating, constipation, anxiety, fatigue, and mood swings, added to the fact that my cholesterol levels were up, I felt like my body was failing me. But I just chalked it up to aging. Perimenopause certainly wasn't on my radar—I didn't even know it existed."

Sara was confused by her symptoms. After all, she ate healthy foods, exercised regularly, and had other worthy habits. Why did she feel so terrible, like she just couldn't muster the energy to be herself? Like so many other people, she approached her doctor with her symptoms. Her doctor told her that it was likely she was getting older, and that the rest of her blood testing looked "fine."

I explained to Sara something that we women are rarely told: Because she was in perimenopause, her symptoms were highly influenced by her gut. If there's anything you get out of this chapter, it's that your gut is a central hub in your body, like the brain. Let's go back to those two commanders using walkie-talkies, sharing crucial information with one another. That's how your gut and brain work together, influencing every aspect of health.

Your gut, which is intricately connected to your hormones, changes throughout your life, especially during perimenopause.

At birth, you receive most of your gut bacteria through your mother's birth canal. Not only do you receive the bacteria from her uterus and vaginal canal but also some fecal bacteria during the process of being born. Infants continue to develop gut bacteria through breastfeeding, the environment, and from other people close to them such as their father or relatives. The first changes occur in infancy, when the gut develops into a digestive and immune system organ. By age 5, the gut has mostly developed into an adult gut and stays that way until we enter perimenopause and menopause, unless we experience a substantial life or dietary change along the way.

As you move into perimenopause, your gut microbiome changes. This happens because some bacteria rely on estrogen, and they die off as estrogen declines. Fluctuations in estrogen and progesterone affect the ecosystem of bacteria in your gut, which can lead to symptoms and health complications. There are more of some bacteria in your gut and less of others. You may suffer vitamin deficiencies because your gut is absorbing nutrients differently. Your cholesterol levels can swing out of range. You get bloated and constipated as hormones begin to alter your gut bacteria. In fact, almost all the symptoms you're experiencing can be traced back to your gut. Unfortunately, most of us are never taught this. One day you might wake up and notice that your body feels different, and without sufficient education or guidance, it feels like the rug has been pulled out from under you.

While these changes to your body may be scary and difficult to manage, you should know that there are many things you can do to actively improve the health of the gut microbiome as you move along the hormonal continuum. It is possible to maintain a healthy gut through diet and lifestyle strategies that optimize your hormones, boost your well-being, and alter the course of your health and your life.

GUT MICROBIOME 101

Your gut is a soft and flexible tube with a unique environment of microbes—100 trillion bacteria, fungi, and viruses to be exact. The gut contains a layer of our cells but has an even thicker layer of cells from these organisms, which serve to protect us. We have 5 to 10 times more of these cells than human cells in our bodies! Collectively, we call this aggregate of microbes the *gut microbiome*.

It is filled with so-called "good" and "bad" bacteria. The good type of bacteria that we get from probiotic foods, for example, is necessary for the biodiversity and overall health of your gut. These "bad" bacteria are things like ultra-processed foods or foodborne pathogens that upend the symbiosis within the gut microbiome. As long as the good bacteria outweigh the bad, you'll enjoy high energy levels, a healthy digestive tract, a healthy body, and a clear, focused mind.

Think of it like a rainforest or coral reef, both very fragile ecosystems like our gut. When too many trees are being cut down or a reef is exposed to higher temperatures, there's an imbalance in the ecosystem that negatively affects the habitats and species that inhabit them. When our gut has an imbalance of bacteria, as in too much bad bacteria, this affects us in tremendous ways from digestion issues, trouble with sleep, mood swings, low energy, and more. The choices we make, such as but not limited to what we eat, determine the balance of the ecosystem within our gut.

The gut has many specific duties: It produces enzymes to break down foods and manufactures vitamins and vital compounds like the feel-good neurotransmitter serotonin or dopamine. In fact, 90 percent of serotonin and other neurotransmitters are produced in the gut. The gut is responsible for the absorption of essential nutrients that are the building blocks for hormones and has a direct relationship with estrogen metabolism.

The gut microbiome is also a major site of thyroid hormone activation (converting T4 to T3). Compromised gut health can lead to the hormone imbalance known as *hypothyroidism*, common in women. It also houses roughly 70 to 80 percent of your immune system and facilitates the elimination of environmental toxins that can lead to symptoms of hormone imbalance.

Believe it or not, the gut communicates with the brain and helps maintain brain health. The master gland in orchestrating hormone production, the pituitary, is in the brain. We'll touch on the mind-gut connection in greater depth later.

The gut has several vital jobs that influence every aspect of your health. So, you can imagine that when your gut has problems and bad bacteria take over, your health will suffer from head to toe and inside and out. One of the biggest problems that becomes more prevalent during perimenopause and menopause is "leaky gut," or irritable bowel syndrome (IBS).

GUT CHANGES DURING PERIMENOPAUSE

To understand leaky gut, think of your gut as a thick, hardy tube that runs from your mouth all the way to your anus. It's pretty resilient, and needs to be, because its job is to keep anything foreign in your digestive tract and out of the rest of the body. Nothing is supposed to get into our organs and blood supply without our immune system saying it's okay.

There are cells lining the intestine, and normally there are tight junctions in your gut that glue these cells to each other. This prevents the contents of the intestine from spilling out into the body without being digested and processed. Unfortunately, these junctions can be damaged by toxins, foods, medications, and stress. The contents of the intestine can then escape into your system. The immune system treats and attacks them like foreign invaders, resulting in inflammation, food reactions, or gastrointestinal symptoms. When food, chemicals, and other foreign matter seep from the gut through compromised junctions, this is called "intestinal permeability," or in layperson's terms, "leaky gut."

When escaping particles get into places where they should not be, this is referred to as "translocation." Translocation makes you more susceptible to chronic inflammation and can lead to a slew of illnesses, including irritable bowel syndrome, Crohn's disease, some cancers, as well as autoimmune and metabolic disorders such as obesity and diabetes. Are you having issues with bloating, indigestion, cramping, or gas? These may also be signs of a leaky gut.

It turns out that hormones are protective of gut problems. Evidence from both animal and human studies indicates that a healthy supply of estrogen and progesterone helps shore up your gut lining and prevent both leaky gut and translocation.

For example, a 2015 lab study published in *The Journal of Trauma and Acute Care Surgery* showed that estrogen protects mucus-producing cells in the intestinal lining against injury.[1] And a 2011 study reported in *American Journal of Physiology-Gastrointestinal and Liver Physiology* using rats and human tissue found that activating estrogen receptors helped reduce translocation.[2] Plus, a 2019 study in pregnant women discovered that progesterone made their gut linings less "leaky."[3]

As these hormones naturally decline while we move along the hormonal continuum, a leaky gut is more likely and translocation more prevalent. With extra work on our nutrition and lifestyle, we can prevent gut problems.

ESTROGEN AND THE GUT-HORMONE CONNECTION

The female gut microbiome is strongly linked to estrogen levels, and we call this association the "gut-hormone connection." As you may already know, estrogen is one of the most crucial hormones involved in the transitions of a woman's life. This hormone regulates blood sugar and lipid metabolism, directs where fat is deposited on the body, helps form bone, and promotes the inflammatory response in the body, among other functions. As estrogen levels go down, the microbiome loses its diversity, increasing the risk of obesity, endometrial cancer, osteoporosis, and cardiovascular disease (I'll go into more detail on the importance of a diverse microbiome on page 75).

Estrogen is also highly involved in the health of your gut microbiome. In fact, there is an entire microbiome solely dedicated to regulating estrogen in your body—the *estrobolome*. (Both men and women have an estrobolome, in case you're wondering.)

The estrobolome is located within the gut microbiome and is comprised of a unique subset of about sixty species of bacteria and fungi that are responsible for metabolizing hormones and regulating the amount of circulating estrogen in your body. The estrobolome makes sure that the amount of estrogen is just right—not too high or too low—and plays a central role in breaking down estrogen, reabsorbing it, facilitating the regulation of estrogen levels, and, consequently, menopausal health.

THE METABOLISM OF ESTROGEN

Before estrogen can reach your gut and the estrobolome, it is metabolized by enzymes in the liver in a process known as phase one and two of estrogen metabolism. Some of the metabolites, or byproducts, of these processes are considered "good" estrogen metabolites. They help regulate normal cell growth triggered by estrogen and prohibit cell division in breast tissue. Other metabolites are considered "bad" in that they can cause damage to cells and DNA and have been linked to an increased risk of breast cancer and other female cancers.

In the liver, the estrogen metabolites are broken down further by a key enzyme called *beta-glucuronidase*, produced by bacteria in the estrobolome. The estrogen either gets absorbed back into the body to be recirculated or gets excreted in your urine or poop—all to support a healthy, ideal balance of estrogen in your body.

The goal of the liver and the estrobolome is to properly break down estrogen into "good" metabolites and to end up with the right amount of estrogen to be recirculated and used in the body. The same thing happens with progesterone or other sex hormones. This process not only maintains hormonal balance but also impacts various aspects of your health, from mood regulation to bone density.

THE PROBLEM OF DYSBIOSIS

A healthy gut microbiome and estrobolome are characterized by a diverse collection of good bacteria. Poor diversity of bacteria, on the other hand, creates "dysbiosis." This means that there are too many of some types and not enough of others. When this happens, the activity of beta-glucuronidase is affected, and estrogen metabolism is impaired.

There are two problems that affect beta-glucuronidase: overactivity and underactivity. You don't want either. Overactivity results in the increased reabsorption of estrogen, or too much circulation of estrogen in the body. These higher levels of estrogen can cause irregular periods, irritability, mood swings, weight struggles, skin problems including acne, bloating and other digestive issues, and other symptoms of perimenopause and menopause. Overactivity is caused by several factors, such as poor diversity of gut bacteria, a diet high in saturated fat, being overweight, smoking, and liver disease.

Dysbiosis can also reduce beta-glucuronidase activity, creating a deficiency of estrogen in the body. Underactivity leads to dry skin, insomnia, urinary tract irritation, mood swings, vaginal dryness, loss of bone density, and other symptoms. Because the microbiome, the estrobolome, and estrogen are so interconnected, many symptoms improve or disappear once you reset your gut.

Quick Pause: Support Healthy Activity of Beta-Glucuronidase

There are many actions you can take right now to support the normal, healthy activity of beta-glucuronidase, an enzyme that's important for regulating estrogen in the body. For example, you can cut back on or avoid alcohol, reduce exposure to toxins in household and personal products, use BPA-free products, and increase your intake of cruciferous and allium vegetables (broccoli, Brussels sprouts, cauliflower, cabbage, radishes, onions, and garlic). These foods support phases one and two for metabolism of estrogen.

You can also support your gut bacteria with probiotics. Supplementation with a broad-spectrum *Lactobacillus* probiotic

---

has been found to help normalize the estrogen metabolism. Additionally, you can try increasing your intake of prebiotic fiber found in fruits and vegetables. Drink green tea; the antioxidant EGCG found in green tea supports beta-glucuronidase. Eat non-GMO organic soy foods. They contain genistein, a phytonutrient that supports beta-glucuronidase. And finally, populate your diet with foods such as oranges, apples, lettuce, and flaxseeds. They contain glucuronic acid, which assists in the healthy metabolism of estrogen.

THE GUT-BRAIN CONNECTION

Besides the gut-hormone connection, there is also a gut-brain connection, as I mentioned earlier. We know, for example, that the brain and gut are literally connected by the *myenteric plexus*—a network of nerve fibers and neuron cells lining our intestinal walls that are influenced by signals from the brain. Like a system of walkie-talkies, gut bacteria are always communicating with the brain and vice versa. In this sense, the gut is an integral part of the nervous system, and the brain can easily influence gut function. The brain-gut connection is so tightly linked that the gut is sometimes called the second brain.

The gut-brain connection is intimately involved in your emotions, which intensify during perimenopause and menopause. In fact, the brain can tell when your gut is inflamed and, in response, triggers feelings of sadness or anxiety. Gut bacteria may also produce molecules that make us crave sugar or feel worried. What's more, dysbiosis and leaky gut can negatively influence neurotransmitters, creating depression, mood disorders, irritability, brain fog, and anxiety.

Many studies have brought to light the importance of this gut-brain axis in health, especially when it comes to mental and emotional symptoms. Recall that most of the feel-good neurotransmitter serotonin is produced in your gut. In addition, certain gut bacteria help with the production of tryptophan, an amino acid that is the building block of serotonin—more on this later.

Further, recent research has found that a beneficial gut bacterium, *Akkermansia*, helps manufacture vitamin B_{12}.[4] This vitamin plays a key role in nerve function; a deficiency of B_{12} is associated with depression, dementia, and poor cognitive function. So, it's becoming evident that good bacteria greatly influence how happy and content you are as well as how clearly you think.

Microbes have the power to affect our emotional health in other surprising ways. One is by manufacturing toxins to make us feel bad or by releasing mood-boosting chemicals to make us feel good. For example, certain bacteria in the *Clostridium* species generate a substance called propionic acid, which can interfere with your body's production of mood-boosting dopamine and serotonin. On the good side, microbes like *Bifidobacteria* help manufacture butyrate, an anti-inflammatory chemical that prevents gut-generated toxins from entering the brain. Other microbes can synthesize the amino acid tryptophan, a building block of mood-lifting serotonin.

Not only that, but gut bacteria affect your stress levels, too—and how well you respond to stress. Research from the UCLA Goodman-Luskin Microbiome Center discovered a fascinating link between our gut bacteria and our ability to cope with stress.[5] The researchers examined more than one hundred adults without mental health problems, assessing their resilience to stress through surveys and MRI scans.

The results were eye-opening. Participants with higher resilience scores, meaning they could better manage stress, also had healthier microbiomes. The researchers attributed this link to the gut-brain connection and the communication flowing bidirectionally between both organs. The brain influences the gut, and the gut impacts the brain. A healthy gut can positively affect brain function, while stress and negative emotions can disrupt the gut, creating a vicious cycle.

Along those same lines, this bidirectionality of the gut-brain connection means that the way you think affects the health of your gut. Studies have shown that people of faith and people who possess a high degree of positivity have healthier guts and more diverse gut bacteria.[6] Maybe you're skeptical, but consider this: When we're happy, we tend to make healthier choices; when we're feeling down, we may make impulsive or unhealthy decisions to help us feel better such as eating sugary foods, consuming alcohol, spending more time looking at screens, or isolating ourselves from friends and family. Further, disturbances in the gut microbiome such as leaky gut or dysbiosis can disrupt the gut-brain connection, bringing on depression, anxiety, and even neurological problems.[7] There's an undeniable relationship between what's happening in the gut and the brain, and it's in our best interest to foster that powerful connection through positive lifestyle choices.

A fascinating study of more than two hundred women by investigators from Brigham and Women's Hospital and Harvard T.H. Chan School of Public Health discovered that there are links between specific gut bacteria and positive emotions like happiness and hopefulness.[8] The key finding was that women who suppressed their emotions had less gut diversity—and were less happy.

The researchers did a second analysis 3 months after the women completed the survey, this time by looking at their stool samples. The team compared those results to the survey responses, looking for connections. Some of the bacteria that turned up in the analysis were linked with health problems, including schizophrenia and heart disease.

These are important findings, with significant implications in perimenopause and menopause when you're experiencing mood swings, depression, anxiety, and poor stress resilience. We need a healthy population of bacteria in our guts to keep us mentally fit. At the same time, how we think, positively or negatively, affects how well good bacteria proliferate in our gut microbiome.

Quick Pause: Reset Your Gut in Just 3 Days

Good news: You no longer have to just "deal with" your symptoms. You can actually change the bacterial makeup in your gut and your estrobolome in a matter of days and feel the effects of this reset quickly as well.

A 2019 study published in the journal *Nutrients* found that a diet rich in vegetables, fruits, and whole grains with a lower intake of red meat, sugar, processed foods, and dairy increased the number of total bacteria in the gut and supported beneficial bacteria like *Lactobacillius* and *Bifidobacterium*.[9] And it happened in just 3 days!

This means you can reset your gut bacteria now and promote its diversity in a very short amount of time—just by choosing the right foods. Before getting into my protocol, let me share some secrets for a gut reset you can start now.

Begin by increasing your fiber. Some great choices for building gut bacteria include fiber-rich foods such as avocados, raspberries, pears, apples, oats and other whole grains, green peas, broccoli, beans, and lentils. Add gut-friendly fermented foods like yogurt, kombucha, kefir, pickles, miso, and sauerkraut.

Then, start each of the 3 days with healthy breakfast foods, like yogurt and a fiber-rich whole grain such as oats. Both ensure that you're looking after your gut.

Continue the rest of the reset with plenty of plant foods. When your body is in hormonal harmony, it is manufacturing hormones, including estrogen, in the correct ratios. It is also metabolizing and eliminating hormones to keep your entire hormonal system humming along. To help support all this, plant foods are a must. They promote healthy estrogen levels by supporting estrogen metabolism. Great choices include dark green veggies, cruciferous veggies, soy foods, brown rice, oats, millet, root vegetables, and seeds.

Proper hydration is super important to keep food moving through your intestines properly, and this movement is vital for a healthy gut. To promote drink-enough-water behavior, stay hydrated throughout the day. Keep a glass or bottle (non-BPA plastic, glass, or stainless steel) of water with you at all times. I also suggest drinking an eight-ounce glass of water every morning and keeping a glass by your bed at night. Drink warm water, too—it takes less time to digest and stimulates digestion while detoxing your system and aiding food through the digestive tract. Drinking warm water is one of the best actions you can take for your health and to help your gut.

A secret way to promote a healthy gut is to get dirty. Let me explain.

In medicine, there is a concept called the "hygiene hypothesis," first proposed in the late 1980s by David P. Strachan, a professor of epidemiology, in *The BMJ*.[10] Strachan noticed that kids in larger households with big families had fewer instances of hay fever. The reason, he hypothesized, was that they were exposed to germs by their older brothers and sisters—and somehow immunized against hay fever. Further research by others discovered that children who were brought up in very clean, highly sanitized environments had higher rates of hay fever, asthma, and a wide range of other conditions.

These observations led to the birth of the hygiene hypothesis. It states that exposure to particular microorganisms (even to germs) protects against diseases by strengthening the immune system. This goes against the grain, though, doesn't it? Honestly, our obsessions with killing bacteria and pristine hygiene habits are doing us more harm than good because they're damaging much of our delicate gut microbiome balance.

Let's compare this concept to building muscle with weights. To build strength and muscle, you must lift progressively heavier weights. If you never expose yourself to heavy lifting, then you'll have a hard time getting stronger. The same can be applied to your immune system, which is what keeps you healthy and helps you heal. To defend against infection, the immune system must be trained by warding off contaminants found in everyday life. If your immune system isn't exposed to contaminants, it will have trouble doing the "heavy lifting" of fighting off infections. The idea is that your immune system needs germs to practice on so that when you're sick or injured, your immune system is ready to fight.

Based on this hypothesis, you can help build a greater diversity of good gut bacteria in your microbiome by getting outside and playing in nature. Why? Dirt contains beneficial bacteria that can boost your gut health. When exposed to dirt, you're exposed to these beneficial bacteria, which can improve your gut health. These microbes train your immune system and make you more resistant to infection. (Along with exposing yourself to dirt, try *not* to over-sanitize!)

Also, when you spend time outdoors, you're exposed to natural sunlight and fresh air. These things can help to reduce stress and improve your mood. Additionally, the act of gardening can be a mindful activity, which can help us focus on the present moment and let go of negative thoughts and emotions.

Warning: Not all bacteria are good bacteria. Playing on the floor of a public restroom is not recommended, for example. It's important in today's world to judge whether our environment is exposing us to good or bad bacteria and to manage risk.

SUPPORT YOUR MICROBIOME AND ESTROBOLOME

Yes, your gut is changing due to perimenopause and menopause, but it is still possible to maintain a healthy microbiome and estrobolome. The food you eat, which becomes the food the critters in your gut feast on, is a crucial component in fostering a diverse microbiome and healthy estrobolome. Of the many lifestyle factors that affect our gut microbes, nutrition is probably the most important.

The strategies to be outlined in this book—ranging from eating a balanced, nutrient-rich diet to incorporating regular physical activity and stress reduction techniques—give you practical ways to enhance the health of your estrobolome. By implementing my protocol, you can not only improve your current menopausal symptoms but also contribute to your long-term health, reducing risks associated with hormonal imbalances such as osteoporosis and cardiovascular disease.

Quick Pause: Fix Bloating Now

Bloating—that uncomfortable feeling of fullness in the tummy, the strange noises, the pain, the sensation of wanting to pass gas—we hate it! Bloating has a variety of causes, ranging from what we eat to medical conditions. Fizzy drinks, beans, broccoli, and cabbage can produce gas during digestion. The gas accumulates in your digestive system, and you bloat. Digestive problems such as constipation and irritable bowel syndrome (IBS) also make us bloat.

Bloating increases during perimenopause and menopause and is sometimes called "meno belly," in which the tummy often pooches out. Besides gas and other causes, blame it also on hormonal changes, such as drops in levels of estrogen due to shifts in the bacterial diversity of the microbiome and estrobolome.

When it comes to bloating, you can wait until it passes or you can take action with some holistic ways to reduce the pain and distention you're feeling. Strategies to help manage bloating include staying active with regular exercise, including yoga. You can chew on fennel seed or infuse it into a tea as a digestive aid, sip ginger or green tea to help ease digestion, and make sure you are drinking enough water throughout the day to keep food moving through your system.

Further, go easy on alcohol and caffeine intake. Both substances can have a detrimental effect on your microbiome health. Follow a fiber-rich, probiotic-rich diet, as outlined in the next chapter, to stop bloating in its tracks. Perhaps most important, limit the amount of processed foods and sugar in your diet, as both of these lead to gut inflammation and worsen bloating.

PART II

Welcome to the Shah Protocol

CHAPTER 5

The 30–30–3 Dietary Framework

I F THERE IS ONE THING you take away from this book, I hope it's the nutrition framework in this chapter—it will change your life within days. Maybe you're thinking, "Yeah, I've heard that before . . ." But I'm not kidding. I'm also not trying to sell you a fancy diet plan. My only aim here is to equip you with the knowledge to fuel your body properly with foods you already enjoy. Nutrition, more than any other aspect of health, gives us the power to unlock our full potential and live better, healthier, more fulfilled lives in ways that extend beyond only the physical. And this isn't just my personal philosophy—it's science.

Sustained proper nutrition is proven to help prevent common age-related illnesses such as diabetes, heart disease, and various types of cancers. The average American diet has high amounts of saturated fats, added sugars, and sodium, and not enough fiber or calcium from whole foods like fruits, vegetables, and grains, making Americans more at risk of obesity, high blood pressure, diabetes, heart disease, cancer, and other health issues.[1] I don't say this to scare you, but I do want everyone to be aware of the pivotal role their diet plays in their aging process and long-term health outcomes.

We live in a world where most people today get the bulk of their information from social media, digital news outlets, and other online sources. It's understandable that people don't want to spend hours combing through medical journals to get their information and instead turn to online figures for guidance, even when that advice is wrong. With so much conflicting information out there about what is considered "healthy," it's hard to know what to believe, where to start, or who to trust. This book is here to help you navigate the often-confusing world of nutrition and aging, break down the science of the hormonal continuum, and give you the tools you need to make decisions about your health with the consultation of your doctor.

What many people don't understand is just how much your gut bacteria play a role in determining how you feel and, further, how everything changes during perimenopause and menopause. When we go through these hormonal transitions, our gut microbiome shifts as our hormone levels change (refer to the previous chapter for a refresher on the science of our gut); we start to lose the gut bacteria that help us take nutrients in from food, that communicate with our brain and with our other hormones, and produce their own neurotransmitters like dopamine and serotonin. These bacteria are amazing and essential for living a healthy life. As you age and hormones like estrogen and progesterone fluctuate and decline, it is crucial that you have ways to keep those bacteria replenished.

It should come as no surprise that the best way to create or modify your healthy gut bacteria is through your diet. Nutrition is king (or shall I say queen) when it comes to changing your gut microbiome. Remember that your gut will respond to diet changes in just 3 days. Gut bacteria need fiber-rich foods, particularly whole foods like fruits, vegetables, nuts, and seeds as well as probiotics so other bacteria can join them. The objective of what we'll call the perimenopausal plate is to:

- Increase, diversify, and support your healthy gut bacteria
- Improve the micronutrients that you're consuming
- Consume more protein to decrease cravings and counteract the muscle loss that occurs during perimenopause and menopause
- Focus on the nutritional value of your food rather than the calorie count
- Make small changes to your diet over time to develop a sustainable and gut-healthy diet in the long term

After having kids and eventually stumbling into what I later realized was perimenopause, I struggled to find a diet that made me feel good and that I enjoyed eating. I tried going low-carb and vegan, but I found that I was buying a lot of processed foods that I didn't feel good about eating. For the longest time, I was eating in a way that I thought would give me the mind and body I had prior to becoming a mother, yet these diets were far from enjoyable, and they didn't make me feel strong in the way that food is intended to. Following many of these trendy diets did not work for me and many other people—that's normal! On a quest to find a diet that I loved and that powered my daily life as a mother and doctor, I went back to basics.

Growing up as a child in India, we always had a lot of nuts such as almonds, pistachios, and peanuts in the house to snack on, and my family's meals were full of vegetables. Daal, a soup made from lentils, was a household staple and is packed with protein, fiber, and magnesium. I've always loved fermented dairy products like yogurt and cottage cheese, which are fantastic sources of protein and probiotics but do not fit under a totally plant-based diet.

I soon realized that the foods I grew up eating were what fulfilled me most, so I ditched the rigid dieting and took a deeper look into the building blocks of nutrition and the brain-gut connection. After tons of trial and error in my own diet- and nutrition-focused research, I developed the 30–30–3 method to promote the foundations of nutrition, improve gut health, manage weight, lower risk of chronic diseases, and even improve mental health. Following this structure was an easy transition that allowed me to eat foods I love without imposing any harsh restrictions or counting calories.

Once I understood the importance of eating a high-protein meal to start the day, I began adding more spices to my breakfasts to make even the simplest plate of scrambled eggs something I looked forward to eating (and a meal that helped boost my fiber while nourishing me with protein). By turning toward my roots and shaping my diet around nourishing foods I love, I'm able to power my day in a way that doesn't make eating feel like a chore, another check off my never-ending to-do list, and that doesn't leave me feeling deprived and struggling with cravings.

Everyone has the right to eat how they feel best fuels them. Though there is nothing wrong with eating low-carb or vegan, trying to follow these rigid diets did not work for my body or lifestyle, and I needed a change. Allow me to introduce you to 30–30–3, a flexible dietary framework I created, designed to fuel your body on your own terms and unlock the best years of your life through nutrition. Let's dive in.

WHAT IS THE 30–30–3?

If you take nothing else from this chapter, take this. Grab a pen, jot down notes as you read, because this new way of thinking about your diet will transform your life. The 30–30–3 is a simple nutrition framework designed to help anyone, regardless of where they are on the hormonal continuum, improve their gut-brain connection through food. Eating "healthy" may look different for everyone, but the goal of the 30–30–3 rule is to cut through the confusion and provide you with a basic structure you can use when planning your meals to ensure you are getting the necessary nutrients each day to optimize your gut, hormone, and brain health.

In our world of fast food, same-day shipping, and 5G internet, we are accustomed to every aspect of our lives being in the express lane, and if we don't get the results we're wanting fast enough, we usually give up and move on. The same goes for nutrition. Maybe you started taking biotin gummies to help strengthen your hair and nails, but after a month you didn't notice any difference, so you didn't buy a new bottle once they ran out, that is, if you finished the bottle at all. Or maybe you tried one of the hundreds of fad diets online promising to shave a few inches off your waist in 30 days but quit after 2 weeks because the meal prepping was just too much on top of everything else you have going on in your daily life. Or maybe you've thought about trying supplements, but you don't know where to begin.

I totally get it—I've been there more often than I like to admit. For us to feel like a lifestyle change is worth it, the change must be attainable every day and give us results we can see or feel within a reasonable amount of time. That's human nature. So many fad diets fail because they are either too overly involved for a normal person with a job and family to integrate, the results are slow-going to non-existent, or they are simply a farce peddled by uninformed figures on social media.

The 30–30–3 is not only easy to incorporate into your diet, but its benefits are almost immediate. We know that improvements to the gut can be felt within days of a dietary change, and the 30–30–3 is designed to achieve just that. I got messages from several patients that following the 30–30–3 changed their life after just a week or two. Within a couple weeks of structuring her diet around getting enough protein, fiber, and probiotic foods, a patient told me she felt like her brain fog was gone and she felt more energized than she had in years. Personally, my mind felt so much clearer once I finally made the switch to focusing on nutrition rather than diet. Once upon a time I was a frazzled mother and doctor blissfully unaware that I was in perimenopause, constantly frustrated at my inability to shake the brain frog that hovered above me like a dark cloud. Now, I'm still in perimenopause, but I'm in full control of my gut and have dialed my lifestyle to support my ever-changing hormones.

Nutrition is powerful, and in my work as a doctor and nutrition specialist, I developed the 30–30–3 to help anyone take back control of their body and unlock their potential through food, just as I have. Let's break it down.

PROTEIN

What if I told you we can set ourselves up for success every day at breakfast through a high-protein meal? I know you've heard that breakfast is the most important meal of the day, but I'm here to tell you that it's true, and here's why. Making a protein-rich breakfast part of your routine improves energy and gut health, and eases the transition through hormonal shifts like menopause. Having adequate protein early in the day stimulates the release of hormones insulin and ghrelin that manage important health factors such as blood sugar balance and hunger levels.

If you implement only one facet of the 30–30–3, it should be setting a target of 30 grams of protein in your first meal of the day. A high-protein breakfast is one of the most underrated ways to improve all the uncomfortable things you're feeling in perimenopause, including poor gut health, weight gain, muscle loss, cravings, mood swings, and more.

Quick Pause: The Deal with Protein

Our gut bacteria love protein, and they help send signals to your brain when you're full, thus curbing those persistent cravings. There's a protein leverage hypothesis that says your body will keep wanting to eat until it gets a certain amount of protein.[2] When you're eating a lot of snacks full of carbs and sugar and not getting enough protein, your body stays hungry and continues to crave more and more.

Diets with low protein intake often lead to overeating and can accelerate muscle loss, especially in middle age. A recent study found that, on average, women lose 1 to 3 percent of their muscle mass every decade until they hit perimenopause, and then it accelerates to 1 to 3 percent per year into menopause and after.[3] Adequate protein intake is crucial during perimenopause since we're already losing a lot of muscle at this stage due to hormonal changes. Along with exercise to combat muscle loss, I cannot stress enough that you want to make sure you're getting enough protein each day.

Protein shakes and bars are okay if they are your only options, but try as much as you can to avoid ultra-processed sources of protein, as these often contain harmful preservatives and high amounts of added sugars. Protein powder manufacturers are not regulated by the FDA, and we do not yet understand the long-term

effects of regular consumption of protein products, many of
which contain heavy metals, BPA, and even pesticides among
other harmful ingredients.[4] When possible, opt for natural,
unprocessed sources of protein to achieve the best outcome
for your gut.

Our first meal of the day is the most important, and we need
to make sure we are fueling our bodies with the right nutrients
not only to start the day but to ensure that we make it through
to dinnertime feeling strong and clearheaded. Whether it be six,
eight, or ten o'clock in the morning, whenever you break your fast
is when you should be aiming for 30 grams of protein.

I understand that 30 grams of protein may sound like a lot, especially for one meal, and maybe breakfast isn't your thing, but I im-
plore you to give this a try in a way that works for you, using foods
that you love. For example, a single egg has 6 grams of protein, so
does an ounce of almonds. A half cup of black beans has 8 grams
of protein, so does roughly 2 tablespoons of peanut butter, and so
does a cup of quinoa, which is rich in fiber. In a 7-ounce container
of Greek yogurt, there are 20 grams of protein, and it counts as one
of your three probiotic foods for the day. There are infinite ways to
achieve 30 grams of protein in a single meal and get your day started
off right. For me, 30 grams of protein looks like scrambled eggs with
cottage cheese, berries, and nuts; or a tofu breakfast scramble packed
with veggies and black beans. If I'm in a rush, sometimes I'll opt for a
protein drink to make sure I'm getting my 30 grams in. Switch it up,
mix in different foods you love, and make a high-protein breakfast
something you look forward to.

The reason I'm emphasizing protein in the morning is because
a high-protein breakfast will kickstart your metabolism for the day
with filling foods so that you aren't struggling with cravings before
lunch or dinner. You can and should absolutely be eating protein
in your other meals as well, but the intention here is to highlight
the importance of protein early in the day—mainly because most
women are not getting enough protein to promote healthy metabolism and cognitive function before beginning their daily routine. It

should be noted that for those with health issues such as kidney disease, a high-protein diet is not recommended. As always, you should consult with your doctor before making any drastic changes to your diet, as it may influence any preexisting health conditions you have.

As a quick note: There is such a thing as too much protein. I know that high-protein foods and protein-dense meals are trending on social media right now, namely in the fitness industry. However, not everyone should be eating tons and tons of protein in every meal. Without knowing your health history, I can't give you a precise daily protein intake recommendation, but in general, healthy women between ages 45 and 65 are recommended between 49 and 90 grams of protein per day. This number, of course, depends on body weight, activity level, and a variety of health factors. Eating too much protein can strain your kidneys and lead to bloating, weight gain, headaches, constipation, brain fog, and increased risk of cardiovascular disease.

I encourage you to measure your current protein intake by examining foods you enjoy consuming on a regular basis. Are you getting enough protein in your first meal? If not, what are some high-protein foods you can incorporate into your first meal of the day to get there? The 30–30–3 method is not meant to restrict the foods you eat, and it is not a rigid dietary plan; 30–30–3 is a flexible dietary framework that helps simplify the most crucial elements of nutrition and promote gut health in a way that can be tailored to any person and diet. Your first 30 grams of protein for the day will likely look very different from mine, and that's okay—that's the whole point! Find what works for you and make it a part of your daily routine. It is my belief that if we lean into what we love, we are more likely to follow through and commit, especially when it comes to food.

FIBER

Around 95 percent of the American population and 75 percent of women have inadequate fiber intake, which is a major issue, because fiber is essential for our gut bacteria to thrive.[5] Most people have no clue that they need to be eating more fiber. The issue of fiber deficits is so widespread and normalized that most people don't realize the extent of prolonged negative effects this deficiency has on their body.

Fiber is the food our gut bacteria need to help reset our hormones and regulate our bowels, and it also makes us feel happy, motivated, and energized. As fiber passes through the body, beneficial bacteria consume it as food, allowing them to become stronger and multiply. With more healthy gut bacteria, we are better protected from disease and harmful germs. Through the process of fiber being broken down in the gut, short-chain fatty acids are produced. As a result, cholesterol and glucose in the blood decrease, which improves metabolism and heart function. Fiber is a valuable input when it comes to your health, and it should not be overlooked. Increasing your daily fiber intake can decrease your chances of heart disease, diabetes, and inflammation in your gut as well as make you feel better mentally and emotionally.

Research has demonstrated that people with fiber-filled diets have less visceral fat, a type of fat associated with many of the common health conditions we see today.[6] In fact, studies have found that when assessing a person's total carbohydrate intake, total fiber intake, glycemic index, glycemic load, and sugar intake, it was the fiber that made the biggest difference to successful aging and lowered health risks.[7]

By starving our gut bacteria of the fiber it needs, we are depriving ourselves of vital nutrients that keep our mind and so many parts of our body going throughout the day. Consuming an adequate amount of fiber diversifies the gut and strengthens the already existing healthy gut bacteria. With these benefits, we are better protected from disease and are more likely to achieve positive health outcomes. If you're struggling with staying alert or having mood swings, consider increasing the amount of fiber in your diet.

This leads me to the second tenet of the 30–30–3 method, which is to get 30 grams of fiber each day. Unlike the first element of this structure, you should space out your fiber intake throughout the course of your day to feed your gut bacteria. In fact, it would be difficult to try and get your full 30 grams of fiber all from one meal. To make hitting that 30-gram target easier, you should be incorporating fruits and vegetables in every meal and in your snacks. I like to use precut or frozen vegetables from the grocery store, which are just as healthy as fresh ones, and they help me save time when preparing meals. Other easy ways to increase your fiber intake is to add nuts to your salads or as a side with your meals, using more spices in your dishes, and introducing more beans or lentils to your diet.

Quick Pause: Polyphenols

Fiber-rich foods like berries, fruits, and vegetables all contain polyphenols, which are beneficial to the good bacteria in your gut. As a bonus, a gene known as "T-bet," found in leafy greens such as broccoli or cabbage, was linked to the production of a particular type of immune cell.[8] These immune cells play an important role in protecting the body from infections entering through the gut. They also help in controlling food allergies, inflammatory diseases, and obesity. The proteins found in green leafy vegetables activate T-bet, and the cells that T-bet activates are known to promote healthy bacteria and heal small wounds common in gut tissue.

As a side note, incorporating thirty different plant foods a week has been shown to improve your gut bacterial diversity, thus improving your overall health. Thirty different plant foods a week sounds like a lot, but that includes seeds, nuts, and spices. Think about how you can add a greater variety of spices to the dishes you already love, maybe try a new vegetable or three, and enjoy the benefits of having a sufficient fiber intake and a diverse gut microbiome.

Of course, fresh is best; but if fruits and vegetables are either too expensive to buy on a weekly basis or if you don't have the time to prepare full meals, there are other ways to make sure you stay on track with eating enough fiber. For example, oatmeal is a great, quick, and inexpensive source of fiber to incorporate into your morning, and popcorn (preferably without loads of butter and salt) is another fiber-rich food that makes for a quick snack throughout the day. While they may take a little more time to prepare, various types of beans like pinto beans, black beans, edamame, and lima beans are all fantastic sources of fiber and are a cost-effective option where a serving of each costs less than a dollar. And as I've said before, get creative with your seasonings—the more spices, the merrier your gut will be.

Quick Pause: Prebiotics

Let's talk about prebiotics. This dietary fiber works to support the healthy bacteria in our gut, or probiotics. A diet containing sufficient prebiotics can help mitigate issues with digestion, bloating, constipation, and can even improve sleep by reducing stress and mood swings. Sources of fiber that are also great prebiotic foods include beans, bananas, whole grains, almonds, leafy greens, garlic, onion, eggplant, artichokes, honey, and more. For women in perimenopause onward, getting enough prebiotics in your diet can promote calcium absorption, improve insulin resistance, promote the reduction of changes to vaginal pH, and help regulate weight. Getting enough fiber is important, but it's equally important that you're paying attention to the types of fiber in your diet. Prebiotics are essential for feeding your healthy gut bacteria and optimizing that gut-brain-hormone connection.

It can be challenging to get 30 grams of fiber throughout the day if you don't have time to eat two or three balanced meals, but I have some tips that can help you stay on track. There are many apps out there such as MyFitnessPal that can help us track fiber. If it's dinnertime and you notice you haven't gotten your full 30 grams yet, maybe add an apple or avocado to whatever you're eating to reach that fiber target. The best way to stay consistent with your diet and to make sure you're getting the nutrients you need is by documenting your food intake in a nutrition or fitness app, using a journal or note in your phone, or to prepare your meals in advance containing all components of the 30–30–3. The first couple of weeks will likely be a bit of a learning curve, especially when it comes to getting enough fiber, but if you commit to yourself and trust the process, I promise your gut and brain will thank you.

PROBIOTIC FOODS

The last piece of the 30–30–3 rule is to eat 3 probiotic foods per day. I know, I know, this may seem a little odd, but let me explain: Probiotic foods have bacteria in them, which heal, strengthen, and create diversity in the gut. Sufficient and diverse gut bacteria send signals to the brain to be happy and energized, and can influence our various personality traits. As we know, gut health and hormone health are closely intertwined; they are connected in a way that, when we take action to improve gut health, hormone health improves along with it. Research shows us that the ingestion of probiotics resulted in significantly lower levels of stress-induced hormones.[9] Probiotics also have a strong influence over the composition of the gut, which balances and supports hormone health overall.

A healthy gut is the greatest response to fluctuating hormones. With it, the body can effectively assess the situation at hand and create what is needed to restore, balance, and soothe symptoms. The influence is remarkable. Studies found that once estrogen is processed by the body, gut bacteria then determine what amount will continue circulating through the body and what amount will be removed through urine and feces.[10]

The immune system benefits greatly from probiotic foods as well, which is a major part of why probiotics are such a staple for longevity that they are considered a potential treatment for inflammatory disease. Probiotics are even linked to decreased anxiety and improved weight management; mental health and weight both have a considerable influence in assessing disease risk and quality of life.

Quick Pause: Eating Probiotic Foods

Many of my patients worry about probiotic foods, thinking that there's no way they could eat 3 servings on top of the 30 grams of protein to start the day and 30 grams of fiber, but let's break it down. A serving of a probiotic food could look like a spoonful of sauerkraut, a tablespoon of apple cider vinegar in water or tea, a serving of probiotic cottage cheese or Greek yogurt, adding fermented vegetables like kimchi to your meals, or having a probiotic beverage like kombucha. Depending on your taste and when you eat, you could even get all three probiotic foods in before noon.

There are so many ways you can get probiotic foods. Your local health food store likely has a refrigerated section with various probiotic options like sauerkraut, kimchi, and sometimes other fermented vegetables like beets. You want to eat 2 full servings a day, which can be broken down into small portions of 3 probiotic foods per day. If all three sources of probiotics are coming from fermented plants, that counts toward your fiber and diversity of gut bacteria!

Remember, your gut microbiome changes as you age, and the decreasing level of bacteria in your gut is why a lot of seemingly inexplicable changes start to happen. It's why you're not able to bounce back from a bad weekend of eating like you used to, why you feel like you always have low energy, why your cholesterol is going up, or why your vitamin D is going down. Your gut health is changing, and one of the best ways you can support it as you move along the hormonal continuum is by eating probiotic foods.

As I've said before, the 30–30–3 is not meant to be restrictive or limit your eating. This framework is here to help you think about what you already eat in a day and introduce reasonable changes to help you make sure your diet is fueling you, making you feel good, and optimizing your gut-brain connection.

Quick Pause: Nutritional Powerhouses

You know what the 30-30-3 is, but what does it look like? Here's a chart that lists some of the best nutrient-dense foods you can incorporate into your diet, if you haven't already. Many of the foods listed here are featured in the recipe section at the end of the book!

Food	Protein (g)	Food	Fiber (g)	Probiotics
Chicken Breast (3oz)	26	Chia Seeds (2 tbsp)	10	Yogurt (with active cultures)
Salmon (3oz)	22	Lentils (½ cup)	8	Kefir
Greek Yogurt (¾ cup)	17	Raspberries (1 cup)	8	Tempeh
Tempeh (½ cup)	15	Black Beans (½ cup)	8	Kimchi
Cottage Cheese (½ cup)	14	1 Artichoke	6.5	Sauerkraut (unpasteurized)
Tofu (½ cup)	10	Avocado (½)	5	Miso
Lentils (½ cup)	9	Broccoli (1 cup)	5	Lassi
Edamame (½ cup)	9	1 Sweet Potato	4	Fermented Pickles
Peanut Butter (2 tbsp)	8	1 Apple	4	Kombucha
Quinoa (1 cup)	8	Brussels Sprouts (1 cup)	4	Apple Cider Vinegar

Almonds (¼ cup)	7	Flaxseeds (2 tbsp)	4	Fermented Cheeses	
Egg (1 large)	6	Blueberries (1 cup)	4	Natto	

WHY 30–30–3?

Believe me when I say the 30–30–3 method is the nutrition hill that I'll die on. Why? Because it works. For everyone. Whether you picked up on it or not, the "perimenopausal plate" doesn't contain any secret woman-only vitamins—it's normal food that anyone can enjoy and benefit from. I frame the 30–30–3 as a dietary framework designed with women in perimenopause at the forefront for its ability to optimize gut and hormone health, but it's something everyone should be doing to live healthier.

Not only did it change my life, making me feel stronger, sharper, and more confident, but it has also helped so many other women already. I've had a patient tell me that her OB-GYN referred her to me for help with her nutrition as she progressed into perimenopause, and I've had other doctors reach out to me saying they mention my name when patients ask about nutrition. This is just the tip of the iceberg. Imagine a world where women everywhere know how to use food to optimize their brain and gut health—imagine how unstoppable we could all be?

The average woman will spend a third of her life postmenopause, and we've been conditioned to think that once we reach that point, our best years are behind us. I'm here to tell you that's just not the case, and you can live life at your fullest potential at any point on the hormonal continuum. My work here is to help women of any age see their power and discover their gifts, and nutrition is our greatest asset in attaining it.

Quick Pause: Getting Started

Any form of dietary change, big or small, can be a challenging process—we are creatures of habit, and it's often difficult to switch from unhealthy foods we enjoy to more nutritious options. I'm not saying you need to scrap your whole diet and throw everything out of your pantry. However, you need to start somewhere, and that somewhere is by looking at the nutritional value of foods you currently eat and reevaluating from there.

At the end of this book, you'll find a protocol for a full 7 days of the 30-30-3 complete with recipes. For now, though, here's a simple chart you can utilize to write down some staples in your diet and visualize their nutritional values. Perhaps you'll notice that you are one of many people in this country living in a fiber deficit. Maybe you're already eating enough protein, but too late in the day. Take a moment to jot down some foods you ate in the past few days and then look up their nutrition facts via tools such as MyFoodData. The goal of this exercise is to help you identify what your nutrition looks like now and what small changes you can make to improve your diet and gut for healthier hormones.

	Food	Protein (g)	Fiber (g)	Probiotic Food Count
Breakfast				
Lunch				
Snack				
Dinner				

Breakfast			
Lunch			
Snack			
Dinner			
Breakfast			
Lunch			
Snack			
Dinner			

Notes

CHAPTER 6

Take-Charge Nutrients

"E AT THIS, DON'T EAT THAT."
"Try this revolutionary workout routine guaranteed to shave three inches off your waist in two weeks!"

"Have you considered the carnivore diet?"

"These gummies will change your life."

"But did you know vegetables cause inflammation?"

"Hollywood's secret to looking 30 at 50 . . ."

You are bombarded with unfounded, unrealistic, outdated, and even harmful misinformation on social media and elsewhere surrounding what you should and shouldn't be putting into your body every day. That's why I'm writing this book. *I'm* here to help *you* wade through the nonsense we see online, decode the science behind nutrition and the hormonal continuum, and prepare you to take charge of your health and your life through informed decision-making. My knowledge and advice are not meant to replace that of your doctor's; rather, the information you gain from this book will empower you to ignore internet fads and strike up important conversations with your doctor about what is right for your body and how you can continue to live life at your fullest potential as you age.

We've talked about how you can use food to optimize your nutrition for promoting your gut-brain connection and minimizing the negative side effects that come with aging and hormonal shifts, but you can also supplement your diet with vitamins and minerals to further boost your health as your body moves along the hormonal continuum.

Spoiler: There is no magical supplement or pill that will suddenly halt the hormonal continuum and keep you 30, flirty, and thriving. And the supple 50-year-old faces we see on the red carpet? Those are thanks to *very* expensive and expertly done cosmetic treatments, despite what some celebrities may claim.

However, even though we cannot stop the clock entirely, there are supplements that can be a game-changer for women across the hormonal continuum including those in the late luteal phase experiencing PMS, women in perimenopause, and more. Having a full and balanced nutrition can help us avoid the more negative or uncomfortable side effects of hormonal transition so that we may age gracefully, Botox or not. While you should strive to get your daily nutrients from your diet, introducing supplements (with your doctor's approval, of course) can be a great way to further enhance the gut, brain, and hormone connection. Supplements are regulated to different standards than those of food or medication, so it's important to always read labels and to discuss with your doctor before introducing any supplements to your routine.

The acronym I want you to remember for this chapter (and others) is MODERN:

M: Magnesium
O: Omega-3s
D: Vitamin D
E: Exercise
R: Rest or sleep
N: Nutrition and Nature

MODERN represents the necessary elements every woman needs to navigate the hormonal continuum through perimenopause and onward. We'll explore more surrounding this idea in a later chapter, but what you need to know now is that what you're putting into your body directly impacts what you're getting out of it, including hormone, gut, and brain health, and your overall longevity.

Quick Pause: Super Nutrients

The supplement that made all the difference for me was magnesium glycinate. Magnesium is a nutrient that is essential for life and helps balance cortisol while raising your levels of serotonin—more on this later. Magnesium glycinate is something that I incorporate regularly in my diet, but I also try to have a high magnesium nutritional plan woven into my 30-30-3 method. Other superhero nutrients you may not have heard about include glucosinolates, polyphenols, phytoestrogens, amino acids, dopamine support foods, omega-3 fatty acids, and all forms of fiber. These are vital nutrients that we can largely get from our diet, and they help protect us from serious illnesses, support our immune system, regulate hunger, increase dopamine, and manufacture hormones.

The meat and potatoes of nutrition science and supplementation can be a little overwhelming to take in; believe me, I've been there. You don't have to tear through this chapter all in one go, because we are going to cover *a lot* about supplemental nutrition and busting myths along the way. Once you've carved out a 30–30–3 plan that works for you, use this chapter as a reference guide to look deeper at your nutrition and locate solutions to help manage your symptoms, whether it's PMS, hot flashes, poor sleep, weight gain, mood swings, or any number of annoying hormone-related side effects you experience each day. Do you feel like you're in a slump and your mood is all over the place? Maybe you're not getting enough vitamin D! Is your diet lacking in important nutrients? Does something just feel *off*? There may be a supplement for that!

In all seriousness, it isn't one size fits all when it comes to supplementation. Take what you need from this chapter and always consult your doctor. Now, make yourself a nice, warm cup of your favorite tea, relax, and prepare to further unravel the not-so-mysterious world of nutrition, what your body needs, and what your body needs less of.

MAGNESIUM

Your body needs more magnesium. Period. It's that simple. There's a reason why everyone and their mother are talking about magnesium and how to supplement it, and that's because it's so incredibly important.

Magnesium is a mineral, naturally occurring in many foods as well as the human body. It is required for energy production and plays an important role in regulating more than three hundred of our body's internal processes, including the regulation of blood sugar, blood pressure, and nerve and muscle function. Magnesium keeps your bones strong and even helps you produce and repair DNA. A diet with sufficient magnesium intake is beneficial for preventing cancer, for chronic inflammation, for brain health, for hormone balance, and for muscle health. There are so many things that magnesium can do, and your body needs it to thrive.

If it isn't already, this mighty mineral needs to be on your nutrition radar. People are not getting enough magnesium in their diet—75 percent of people, that is.[1] More specifically, women, especially those in the menopausal transition, tend to suffer from low levels of magnesium. For this reason, increasing magnesium intake through supplements or food is a wonderful first step for resetting hormonal balance and reaping the benefits a nutrient-balanced diet can offer.

Quick Pause: Magnesium Magic

Let's break it down. For every 100 grams of magnesium you eat, you have a drop of 24 percent in pancreatic cancer risk.[2] A person with a diet that incorporates the highest recommended intake of magnesium, which is 550mg per day, could have a 40 percent decreased risk of all-cause mortality and a 50 percent decrease in cancer mortality.[3] Magnesium also helps the brain grow and prevents dementia. Seriously. Adding more magnesium to your diet is an easy change you can make now that will have tremendous benefits for the rest of your life.

While this chapter is about how to supplement with vital nutrients, note that you should be getting most of your vitamins, minerals, and nutrients from your food. Magnesium-rich foods include pumpkin seeds, almonds, cashews, chia seeds, spinach, avocado, and edamame, to name a few. Nuts, seeds, beans, and leafy greens are all great sources of magnesium that can easily be woven into your 30–30–3 plan if you're not already eating them. If you already eat these foods, congratulations! You're on the right track. Supplementing with additional magnesium can help get you to the recommended dose of 550mg each day if you need it.

Quick Pause: There Are Different Types of Magnesium?

Not all forms of magnesium are created equal. While increasing your magnesium intake is a must, magnesium oxide, a salt commonly sold in powder or capsule form, has a low absorption rate, meaning it won't do much for you if your goal is to increase your daily magnesium. If you decide taking supplements is right for you, be sure to read the labels before purchasing so you know what you're getting. Taking magnesium oxide won't hurt, but it also won't provide you with the same benefits as other forms of magnesium with higher absorption rates.

As I mentioned before, magnesium glycinate made a huge difference in my life. It didn't take long after introducing it into my diet in the evenings before I noticed I was getting more restful sleep, and my anxiety felt like less of a weight over my head. Magnesium glycinate is easily absorbed into the digestive tract and has been shown to promote better sleep, protect against heart disease and diabetes, and has calming properties that can be helpful for mental health issues such as depression, anxiety, stress, insomnia, and others. Magnesium glycinate, for me, has been nothing short of a life saver. It's a great supplement for women in menopausal transition, but it is also something that anyone can get tremendous benefits from.

A better option for those looking to supplement magnesium but are sensitive to constipation or GI issues is magnesium citrate. It's a form of magnesium bound with citric acid that has natural laxative properties and similar calming effects as magnesium glycinate. Magnesium threonate is another great supplement option with a high absorption rate and it promotes brain health. This form of magnesium is shown to cross the blood-brain barrier to improve memory, and it can even help treat disorders like depression and Alzheimer's. Magnesium glycinate and threonate are my preferred supplements for anxiety, a boost in serotonin, and sleep; these can be taken together to maximize the benefits across different aspects of health.

I take magnesium threonate in the morning and magnesium glycinate in the evening before bed, and I've found that this combination really works for me. Through this small change in my routine, I've been able to transform my sleep and the way I feel with my hormones. Do some experimenting and take a closer look at your diet to estimate how much magnesium you're already getting through foods (like the chart at the end of the previous chapter) before making the decision to introduce a supplement. Increasing your magnesium intake is a small and simple change you can make that will have tremendous long-term benefits as your hormones shift through the hormonal continuum.

Quick Pause: Cortisol-Reducing Supplements

Supplements designed to reduce cortisol levels have been all the rage across social media for good reason. People are overworked, constantly stressed about a myriad of things, and these issues have only intensified since the pandemic. The National Study of Daily Experiences (NSDE) found that adults younger than 30 experienced the greatest and most frequent levels of stress (and reactivity), but that these stress levels and occurrences declined steadily over the course of the next 20 years.[4] They found that adults age 54 and older experienced lower baseline stress and maintained relatively stable stress reactivity for the duration of the 20-year study.

These findings from the study reflect the trajectory of our hormones as we move along the continuum as well: Our sex hormones are at their peak before and around the age of 30 and then begin to gradually decline until we settle into a plateau with lower estrogen. Cortisol is a hormone, and when we are stressed, the brain's hypothalamus tells the adrenal glands to release cortisol. If you've ever experienced a strong feeling of panic, like fight or flight, that was your brain releasing high amounts of cortisol to face a perceived threat. The problem, however, is that our brain cannot filter out the types of stress we experience daily. The brain is biologically wired to release cortisol in response to stress, such as being chased by a bear, protecting a loved one from danger, or hunting for food.

Seeing as though the average person doesn't experience life-threatening circumstances on a daily basis, our brain registers other stressors like giving an important presentation at work, planning a wedding, driving in rush-hour traffic, grocery shopping in Trader Joe's at 6 p.m. on a Monday, accidentally liking your ex's Instagram post from four years ago, and forgetting to pay a credit card bill as high-stress events, thus triggering the release of cortisol based on our strong reactions to events that are, relatively, low-stress in nature. Too many of us go through life chronically stressed, and it's hurting our health. Enter cortisol-reducing supplements.

Supplements that have the effect of reducing cortisol levels include magnesium, vitamin D, ashwagandha, omega-3 fatty acids, CBD, ginseng, and L-theanine, among others. While there's still a long way to go in understanding the long-term effects of various supplements on cortisol levels, there's evidence that supports taking supplements outside of our diet to decrease cortisol.[5] We know that magnesium, omega-3s, and vitamin C help lower cortisol as well as support other functions in the body, but you may want to consider options like CBD, ginseng, L-theanine, and ashwagandha with the help of your doctor. If you struggle with chronic stress, perhaps there are supplements (rather than medications) you can incorporate to balance your cortisol naturally.

VITAMIN D

Vitamin D is ubiquitously low in women in perimenopause. In fact, nearly every woman whose levels I've ever checked has been vitamin D deficient. Why is this? While there's no blood test that can tell you where you are in your journey toward menopause, low vitamin D levels are a strong indicator that you're experiencing hormonal shifts and progressing along the continuum either through perimenopause or menopause.

During perimenopause, our microbiome is changing, and the way we absorb nutrients changes as well. There isn't a ton of research on why perimenopause causes vitamin D levels in particular to drop, and we don't fully understand why this happens, but it is no secret that vitamin D deficits are an issue across the board for women in perimenopause and menopause. Approximately 70 percent of all menopausal women are vitamin D deficient; one of the negative side effects of menopause is the body's reduced ability of the skin and kidneys to produce vitamin D as well as the intestines' reduced ability to absorb vitamin D, further exacerbating the issue.[6]

Quick Pause: More Vitamin D, Please

Did you know the official NIH recommended daily amount of vitamin D per day is roughly the same for women who are 19 and women who are 70?[7] You may be thinking, "What?" It's as bizarre as it sounds. The recommended 600 IU (15 mcg) of vitamin D for women reflects someone who doesn't have a vitamin D deficiency, yet *we know* that women in perimenopause onward more than likely are vitamin D deficient. My recommendation for women in perimenopause onward is to get 2000 IU of vitamin D per day; of course, it's always smart to get your vitamin D level checked by your doctor in case you are not deficient enough to warrant supplementation.

If we know that women's vitamin D levels drop as they move along the hormonal continuum, why are doctors still recommending them the same vitamin D intake as a 19-year-old? That answer in itself could be a book. The greater health community neglects to consider that women experience gradual and continual decreases in vitamin D in accordance with drops in estrogen and therefore need additional vitamin D to make up for what was lost. It is, unfortunately, all too common that aspects of women's health are vastly misunderstood and misrepresented in medical literature as well as the media. I wake up each day with a purpose to do my job and empower women, to equip them with the knowledge they need to optimize their health, so that every woman feels she can take charge of her life and live at her full potential—at any age.

When a patient comes to me not sure of where she is on the hormonal continuum or if she is struggling with common perimenopause symptoms, one of the first things I'll do is check her vitamin D levels. And as I've said, most of the patients I see are in fact vitamin D deficient. My recommendation to these women is to increase their vitamin D to 4000 to 5000 IU per day, perhaps even more for those with a severe deficiency. I'm here to bust the myth once and for all that the recommended vitamin D intake is the same for teenagers as it is for women in perimenopause. That's just absurd. It ignores the many fundamental changes women experience as their hormones transition toward menopause. Vitamin D is so very important, and this only proves to be more essential as we age.

During my immunology fellowship, vitamin D was the "vitamin of the year" because it does so much for our immune system. Research shows that many of the body's organs and tissues have receptors for vitamin D, which tells us that having an adequate amount of it is important for balance and maintaining health. Vitamin D promotes the absorption of calcium for bone production and calcification, playing a pivotal role in preventing osteoporosis. Additionally, vitamin D's anti-inflammatory and antioxidant properties are what stimulate improvements in muscle function, immune health, and cognition. This is why improvements in hormone function are associated with increased amounts of vitamin D.

Quick Pause: Calcium and Vitamin D

Let's take a moment to talk about calcium. You already know that we need calcium to keep our bones and muscles strong; however, did you know that our bodies need vitamin D to absorb that calcium? As we transition into perimenopause and our vitamin D levels drop, we also experience a decreased ability to absorb calcium, which contributes to the prevalence of a loss of bone density and osteoporosis among women older than 50. However, I don't recommend a calcium supplement, and here's why: Taking too much calcium can lead to calcium deposits in your arteries and put you at greater risk of heart disease. Also, there isn't a clear recommended daily intake for calcium across the board, as your ideal intake will differ from that of someone older or younger than you, or someone with a high risk of cardiovascular disease, and so on.[8] Instead, you can help address a calcium deficiency through increasing your vitamin D, which will help your body absorb the calcium you get from your diet naturally. If you are curious about whether a calcium supplement is right for you, consult your doctor for an accurate assessment.

We get vitamin D from sunlight and our diet, and we can also supplement with it in the form of vitamin D_3. Sunlight resyncs the circadian rhythms in your brain and body. We have a master clock in our brain, and we have clocks all over our body in every single organ.

When we get sunlight or natural light, it serves as a reset that tells the body, "Okay, it's morning," which tells the brain, and the brain ends up telling all the peripheral clocks around the body what time it is.

Everything in your body works on circadian rhythms. You'll want to prioritize getting natural sunlight and supplementing with vitamin D to get your levels out of that decreased estrogen-induced deficit not only for the vitamin D benefits but also for circadian rhythm benefits. It's really important to have alignment with the time of day and your circadian clock, because when your circadian rhythm is misaligned, you experience heightened anxiety or depression and can have injuries.

Soak up the sun (wear sunscreen, of course)! Your body needs it. Even if it's not a clear, blue-sky day, you can still access the benefits of vitamin D by being outside. Take every opportunity to squeeze in time outdoors! Few foods naturally offer vitamin D. However, sunlight triggers a chemical conversion in the skin in which the body creates vitamin D. While the body's ability to produce vitamin D is reduced during perimenopause and menopause, getting outside and enjoying sunlight as much as possible will help keep you from living with a vitamin D deficiency and help combat bone density loss among other negative outcomes.

Having adequate vitamin D promotes better vaginal health, bone density, mood, and hormonal transition. I often say that vitamin D acts more like a hormone in the body than a vitamin due to its ability to help control the functions of cells and organs. It's like hormone therapy without hormone therapy. If you aren't quite sure where you are on the hormonal continuum, go get your vitamin D levels checked. If they are low, consider it a sign that your hormones are shifting, it's likely you are in perimenopause, and you need to start getting more sun and supplementing with vitamin D_3.

OMEGA-3 FATTY ACIDS

Omega-3s are another trendy buzzword nutrient on social media right now, so let's break down what they are and why we need them. Omega-3 fatty acids are a form of healthy polyunsaturated fat that your body needs to support various functions. There are three different types of omega-3s: DHA and EPA both come from marine life, and ALA comes from plants. Omega-3s are responsible for maintaining the health of our cells by protecting cell membranes and interactions between cells as well as providing energy for our cardiovascular and endocrine systems.

Quick Pause: The Scoop on "Bad" Fats

A well-known benefit of omega-3 fatty acids is their ability to lower high triglyceride levels. Triglycerides are another form of fat that comes from foods like butter, fatty meats, cheeses, whole milk, and more—these can be saturated or unsaturated depending on the molecules' bonds. A diet reliant on foods containing high amounts of triglycerides, saturated fats, sugars, simple carbohydrates, and trans fats (the type of fat found in artificial or processed foods) puts you at greater risk of a slew of health problems, not to mention it totally derails the balance within the gut microbiome. We can think of triglycerides in excess as "bad" fats, whereas omega-3s are "good" fats. When our triglyceride levels are too high, we are at greater risk of pancreatitis, stroke, and cardiovascular diseases.

If you're thinking, "This sounds like cholesterol," you would be right—well, sort of. Triglycerides and cholesterol are both types of these fatty substances called *lipids*. However, triglycerides are a fat, and cholesterol is a protective, waxy substance produced in the liver. Despite its often negative connotation, cholesterol in itself is not inherently bad. In fact, cholesterol is what helps fortify cell walls and protects our nervous system, and it aids in the digestion process as well as the production of certain hormones. We need cholesterol (and triglycerides) to live, but problems arise when those levels get too high.

Apart from diet, there are several factors that contribute to dangerously high triglyceride levels such as a sedentary lifestyle, excessive alcohol consumption, smoking, and thyroid, kidney, and liver diseases. Women in perimenopause are actually more likely to have higher triglyceride levels at this stage due to a drop in estrogen and changes in how fat is distributed throughout the body.[9] Maintaining a healthy lifestyle consisting of a good diet–ahem, the 30-30-3–and regular exercise will help you keep those triglycerides in check, but it is also a good idea to have your doctor perform routine blood tests to monitor lipid (cholesterol and triglyceride) levels.

The internet is rife with information, accurate and otherwise, on "good" and "bad" fats. The carnivore diet, for example, is inherently high in triglycerides and therefore an incredibly harmful diet for many people, including women in perimenopause. I don't bring up triglycerides to scare you but rather to call attention to an aspect of health and nutrition not often spoken about in popular media. The more knowledge you have of the inner workings of your body and the impacts the food you eat have on biological processes, the larger positive influence you can have on your long-term health outcomes. Plus, you'll be able to spot misinformation online and share what you know with others.

A recent study in *The American Journal of Clinical Nutrition* found that long-term supplementation with omega-3s DHA and EPA can lower one's risk of developing Alzheimer's disease, dementia, or other forms of cognitive decline.[10] While research is still ongoing, omega-3 fatty acids may be beneficial in the perimenopause to menopause transition by decreasing symptoms such as hot flashes, joint pain, PMS pain, and even treat or prevent conditions like major depressive disorder and osteoporosis.[11] There have even been studies that found smokers with a high omega-3 level had the same risk of heart disease if not less than nonsmokers with a low omega-3 level.[12] Now, this study is not saying that smoking is healthy, but rather it demonstrates the vast potential of health benefits from increasing your omega-3s, that even those with unhealthy lifestyle choices can improve their health through omega-3 supplementation. We still have much to learn about the benefits omega-3s have for supporting women through the hormonal continuum, and I encourage you to ask your doctor if adding it into your routine could be right for you.

We've talked about strengthening the gut-brain connection through our diet, but another element essential in achieving this balance is through exercise. Technically, exercise is not nutrition, but it goes hand in hand. Exercise plays a key role in how the gut bacteria communicate with the brain.

Rather than waste your time by reiterating the long and arduous lectures from my time in medical school, I'll give you the cheat sheet on short-chain fatty acids:

When you exercise, the gut bacteria we learned about in the previous chapters get super happy and they produce these magical compounds called short-chain fatty acids (SCFAs). SCFAs go to your brain, calm the inflammation, and make it happier and healthier. They also go all over the body, sort of like anti-inflammatory magic fairy dust. While our body can produce SCFAs, we cannot produce the amount of omega-3 fatty acids we need to survive. Instead, we get these from our diet or through supplementation.

So, you decide that you want to get more SCFAs. How? You exercise, you eat fiber, you eat foods that have good bacteria, and they produce short-chain fatty acids. You should also consider supplementing with omega-3 in the form of fish oil, flaxseed oil, or another variation of EPA, DHA, and ALA. These are essential if you want to improve your mood, your health, and lower inflammation in your body.

Quick Pause: The Inflammation Myth

Let me quickly bust another myth for you: Inflammation is not bad.

When you're sick, a virus enters your body, or you get injured, your brain triggers the immune system to send out inflammatory cells and cytokines, which stimulate the production of more inflammatory cells. This process is what's referred to as *acute inflammation*. You can think of things like bruises and fever as by-products of acute inflammation; basically, these momentarily painful things we experience after triggering an immune response are signals that the immune system is actually working. Think about it–if you fall and get hurt, you want your body to heal and fix it. That healing process involves a degree of inflammation in order to recover from the injury. A body without inflammation is a body that cannot heal itself.

What we don't want is chronic inflammation. We want something to go around the body, like short-chain fatty acids, and heal some of the inflammation we are experiencing due to exercise, minor injuries, or overexerting ourselves in some way. It's crucial to understand that inflammation is not all bad and that we need to produce more anti-inflammatory compounds in our body naturally. This can be accomplished through eating more anti-inflammatory compounds in our food so that we can calm the chronic burning inflammation in our bodies, especially as we get older. If you feel like you're constantly inflamed no matter what you do, consult your doctor about how to address it.

MAXIMIZING NUTRITION: BEYOND THE BASICS

Now that you've got the basics down, let's take this a couple of steps further and talk about other ways to maximize your nutrition to best support you on the hormone continuum.

POLYPHENOLS

In the previous chapter, I mentioned that your fiber-rich foods like fruits, berries, and vegetables all contain polyphenols, which help nurture good bacteria in your gut. But there's more. Polyphenols are a naturally occurring micronutrient and powerful antioxidant found in plants that can work to prevent or even reverse damage to your cells caused by aging. And the best part? You don't need to supplement these in your diet because there are over eight thousand types of polyphenols found in the foods you are already eating.

A diet full of foods rich with polyphenols is shown to boost your immune system and reduce your risk of chronic conditions such as diabetes, certain types of cancers, heart disease, and chronic inflammation. Studies have found that getting more than 650mg of polyphenols per day can greatly decrease your risk of disease and death and give you more of the best days of your life.[13] Along with fresh plant-based foods, you can get your polyphenols from herbs, nuts, olives, dark chocolate, coffee, tea, and even small amounts of red wine.

Quick Pause: Super Foods, For Real

Let's talk about the nutritional powerhouse that is a blueberry. Blueberries are amazing in their ability to improve mood, cognition, and protect against dementia. One cup of blueberries a day is enough to spark these changes. In fact, recent studies show that 1 cup of blueberries almost instantly, within an hour, makes you smarter.[14] That is, eating blueberries increases alertness and promotes healthy cognitive function with near-immediate effects. I mean, if you're not blown away by this, I don't know what else I can tell you. But things like blueberries have polyphenols and fiber. Nutrient-rich foods like blueberries, which are not processed at all, can help you in big ways that we're just understanding now.

Another game changer is cacao powder or cocoa powder, and some dark chocolate. Eating 1 tablespoon per day of unprocessed cocoa powder for 12 weeks was shown to increase muscle strength. Imagine that you could increase your muscle strength and mass by just one spoonful of cocoa powder a day. Crazy, right? You may have heard of the Guna people of Panama, an Indigenous matriarchal society whose people are known to be extremely healthy, live longer, and have remarkably low blood pressure and pristine cardiovascular health. One reason for this is that their diet is full of high-flavonol foods, such as unprocessed cocoa, which they soak in water and drink on a regular basis.[15] Dark cocoa can also improve vascular stem cells by 50 percent, and it actually improves heart health as well.[16] Cocoa powder is incredibly versatile: You can make it into a drink, you can add it to your foods, you can make it into a pudding, or you can have it in your desserts.

Now, I'm not talking about getting a whole bunch of candy bars and claiming you're eating them for your brain health. The problem with cocoa, unlike blueberries, is that it's often processed with lots of milk and sugar. And even for me, it's sometimes hard to differentiate between healthy cocoa and unhealthy cocoa products. The best way to do it is to use unprocessed dark cocoa powder in your cooking, think 100 percent or 80 percent, in your baking or in your drinks, because it's really hard to find high-quality dark chocolates that achieve this effect.

If you're thinking, "I need my chocolate fix now. What should I buy?" here are some brands I recommend at your nearest grocery store: Theo Chocolate, Hu Kitchen, Endangered Species Chocolate, Navitas Organics, Raaka, and Beyond Good. There are some great generic brand options out there as well; just take a look at the packaging for the sugar content before buying.

You shouldn't be taking a supplement to get your 650mg of polyphenols per day since you should be getting them through your diet. However, if you think you may not be getting enough with your current diet, introducing more foods like blueberries and cacao can be a great way to help you get there.

Quick Pause: Starch Hack

Carbs. We love them, but they don't often love us back. A diet heavy in carbs can cause unwanted weight gain and bloating, and spike your blood sugar. I love bread and pasta as much as the next person, and I'm going to share a little secret that allows me to get plenty of carb-filled foods without all the negative consequences of doing so.

There is a way to naturally alter the caloric and nutritional value of your favorite carbs overnight. Take the bread you use for toast in the morning, cooked pasta you prepped for tomorrow's dinner, or the rice you cooked last night and put them in the freezer or refrigerator. During the cooling process, the starch in these foods converts to resistant starch. Resistant starch is better for gut health than nonresistant starch; it makes you feel fuller despite being less calorie-dense, and it won't contribute to spikes in blood pressure. As a bonus, it will increase the shelf-life of your groceries.

Remember, carbohydrates are essential for their role in driving tryptophan across the blood-brain barrier (BBB), protecting our brain from toxins in the body. "Carb" doesn't have to be a dirty word, and there are tons of ways to enjoy these foods guilt-free. When you're ready to eat those frozen foods, just thaw and cook as normal. Apart from being a gut-health hack, freezing ready-made foods is an awesome meal-prep hack and timesaver as well.

THE TRUTH ABOUT COFFEE

There is much discourse surrounding coffee and how it impacts our health. I'm here to tell you that up to 3 cups of coffee a day is found to be protective for longevity and brain health.[17] Consider this permission to ignore the naysayers out there telling you to ditch your morning pick-me-up. Coffee, in itself, is not bad for you, and I give it the Dr. Amy Shah stamp of approval.

Tea is also shown to be beneficial to your health and decreases mortality, whether it be green, black, oolong, chai, or any other variety. Three cups a day can actually decrease your mortality by 24 percent, and within an hour after consuming tea, you see genoprotective effects.[18] It lowers DNA damage and is full of antioxidants, especially green tea. Black tea also has antioxidants that can be protective for your brain, heart, and DNA.

If there's one thing my friends and family know about me, it's that I'm an absolute chai fanatic. Growing up in a Southeast Asian household, my parents made chai for me from school-age onward, and I've been a huge chai consumer ever since. I even created a healthier version of chai that I sell on my website, without the typical sugar and processed dairy. The polyphenols in chai, or any tea for that matter, make it a central part of my morning routine. Chai is something I look forward to every day, and it's also great for my health and longevity.

Coffee has very similar effects on our body as tea. It's great for our brain and also cuts mortality risk.[19] But you might be thinking, "I heard that in perimenopause you are more sensitive to caffeine?" Great point. Caffeine can be really, really difficult to tolerate in perimenopause. In fact, I can't have caffeine after noon. So how do you reconcile this data about tea and coffee? How can it be good for you but also bad for you? It's simple. I recommend having your tea and coffee in the morning, and not necessarily first thing—wait until an hour after you wake up—and then stopping at noon. That might be a very small window for some of you, but hear me out.

When you have caffeine in the morning, it helps you become and stay alert, and it will help you with genome protective effects. It has antioxidant properties, and having it in the morning won't affect your sleep or increase anxiety. You may be wondering why I recommend waiting an hour before you have your caffeine in the morning. Well, having caffeine first thing can disrupt the regulation of adenosine and cortisol levels and actually cause you to crash harder once that caffeine wears off. Adenosines are nucleosides in cells that play vital roles in the processes of energy transfer and sleep regulation, for example. Adenosine levels in the brain are at their lowest upon waking, build during the day, and then decrease while you sleep. They're one of the ways our body knows when it's time to rest. Inversely, cortisol levels are at their highest upon waking and then gradually decrease throughout the day. Caffeine acts as a block to adenosine, which in theory should prevent us from getting tired. However, if you block the adenosine too early, such as 30 minutes after waking up, you won't be able to capitalize on the benefits of cortisol being at its peak and your natural alertness, and this also means you will feel way more tired midday, when your cortisol is in decline and adenosine levels increase. This *does not* mean to keep drinking caffeine later in the day to compensate for your drop in energy. Blocking adenosine later in the day means you will experience difficulty falling asleep and potentially feel even groggier the next morning. So, if you're someone who really suffers from a post-coffee slump, wait to have your first source of caffeine for about 60 to 90 minutes from the time you wake up.

Quick Pause: Caffeine and Sleep

For those of you who are sensitive to caffeine, in perimenopause, having trouble sleeping, having anxiety issues, having heart palpitations, or experiencing other symptoms associated with caffeine, stop having caffeine about 10 hours before bed. That may mean stopping at 11 a.m. or noon.

Once I figured this out, there was no going back. And this doesn't mean that I must avoid coffee meetups with friends in the afternoon–I just opt for decaf instead of the full-caf version. (Remember, decaf does have a little bit of caffeine, but it won't impact you as much as the fully caffeinated products.) If you are someone who doesn't need or drink caffeine, that's okay (and lucky you!). Decaffeinated tea, like green or herbal teas, have some of the same benefits as a caffeinated version. (The protein chai I created is decaffeinated, and it's a great afternoon treat for when I want something that tastes great and makes me feel good without keeping me awake for hours after bedtime.)

Coffee drinkers between the ages of 40 and 69 have a 14 percent lower risk of dying over a 10-year period, and despite the rumors about coffee being detrimental during the perimenopause and menopausal transition, 1 to 3 cups a day is shown to be perfectly fine for you, healthy even.[20] Remember, it's the nutritional powerhouses like polyphenols and antioxidants, not the caffeine and certainly not the sugar, that make coffee and tea great staples in your routine. Go forth and enjoy your morning cup of caffeinated bliss every day if that's what makes you happy. Just be cognizant of when you're consuming caffeine and when you plan to go to sleep, and refrain from loading up your drink with processed sugars, syrups, and creams.

PROCESSED FOODS AND SUGAR

I've given you an abundance of advice, tips, and tricks to better your nutrition, but to optimize your brain, gut, and hormone connection, there are some things you need to avoid, too. More than 60 percent of the American diet today consists of ultra-processed foods.[21] These are foods that could never be re-created in a kitchen—they have to be manufactured using unnatural chemicals and ingredients to exist. When I talk about ultra-processed foods, I'm talking about sugary drinks, bags of chips, candy bars, packaged baked goods, things with artificial food coloring, and so much more. Beyond being ultra-processed and wholly unnatural, these foods are not normal sources of fuel for humans, and our body does not know what to do with them.

Prepackaged snacks, fast food, and sugar take a massive hit on our gut microbiome. Ultra-processed foods are convenient and overwhelmingly available, and many of us are unaware of how our bodies are responding to this type of diet. Through clever marketing and societal acceptance of these foods, we have been conditioned to believe they are the norm, that they are okay and safe to eat. Now, we crave these ultra-processed foods because our gut bacteria are hooked on them, and as a result we have unbalanced hormones from what should be providing us with nutrition.

Let me reiterate: This is not normal.

The food industry engineers foods to keep us coming back for more. Ultra-processed foods target the brain's reward center and flood it with pleasure signals that intensify cravings. Science tells us that high-glycemic foods in particular trigger the brain's reward centers. The glycemic index (GI) charts the impact a certain food has on raising our blood sugar levels. The higher the glucose level, the quicker the increase. The strategy that helps food manufacturers achieve this surge is known as the *bliss point*; it is an intense combination of sugar, fat, and salt that stimulates the reward and pleasure centers in our brain.[22] This type of pleasure experience resembles addiction and keeps people coming back for more rather than turning to natural, whole food options.

Simply put, ultra-processed foods are toxic to the body; eating a diet made up of primarily processed food can cause chronic inflammation, depression, anxiety, a long list of diseases, and premature death. My warning against processed foods extends beyond women in perimenopause—this is important for your friends, family, and children, too. The average American teenager eats a diet of 75 percent processed foods. I am a mother of two teenagers, and I see how much processed foods are a part of their lives, woven into the fiber of culture and friend groups.

Teenagers getting their first taste of freedom, whether it be at school or with their friends, turn to tasty, convenient, cheap foods and snacks. This behavior becomes habit over time and carries over into college and adulthood. Studies upon studies have identified links between ultra-processed foods and poor mental health. These seemingly tasty foods are not worth the sinister mental and physical risks for you or your children.

Quick Pause: Liquid Calories

In talking about ultra-processed foods, it's also important to note the prevalence of ultra-processed, sugary drinks and the negative impacts that come from these liquid calories. Drinks with added sugars like sodas, juices, flavored coffees, and alcoholic beverages are all ways that you unknowingly drive up your glucose levels. The glucose spikes from sugary drinks increase bad inflammation and contribute to worsening mental health. People with a reliance on sugary, processed beverages in their daily life are found to have the worst mental health.[23] There is absolutely a link between the types of food–nutrients–we put into our body and our state of mind.

Before introducing supplements to your diet, before doing anything else, you need to decrease the amount of ultra-processed foods you're consuming in a day. Making that change alone will improve your menopausal symptoms, as well as decrease your risk of death. For every 10 percent you decrease your ultra-processed food consumption, you get a 14 percent decrease in your risk of mortality.[24] Cutting out ultra-processed foods will not only make you feel better, but it will also extend your life. This is step one.

Getting rid of ultra-processed foods and opting for whole and natural choices can be a difficult process. After all, these foods were intentionally designed to keep us hooked. The trick is to identify your cravings and look for healthy alternatives that are equally as satisfying and filling. Even with this style of thinking, it's almost impossible to eliminate processed foods entirely.

Now apply what you've learned about our gut microbes. The more we increase the natural foods we eat and decrease the number of processed foods in our diet, the stronger and more plentiful our healthy bacteria become. When we regularly consume unnatural foods, we surrender our full capacity of choice due to their addictive nature.

A balanced diet does not rule out foods high on the glycemic index (a scale from 0 to 100 used to measure how quickly a food spikes blood sugar levels), but being aware of what falls into this category, what's actually in the food products you regularly add to your shopping list, can help with portion control and disease prevention. Foods with a low GI break down slower and may help with feeling fuller, longer. I promise, your body will be more satisfied when you try to eat more nutrient-dense foods. In time, you will overcome the manufactured bliss point cravings and be less inclined to reach for processed and gut-damaging foods.

A huge component of why ultra-processed foods, and some un-processed foods, are so bad for you is due to sugar. We all love sugar, but it does not love us back. Sugar is an inherently addictive ingredient because of the way it influences the brain's reward system, making us feel hooked. Ultra-processed foods are largely high in sugar, meaning they are high-GI foods that will cause dramatic spikes in blood sugar. Diets high in sugar are a massive stressor on our gut and overall health.

High-fat, high-sugar diets are typical in the West—and this is a problem. Studies found that after 4 weeks of this type of diet, the microbiome is significantly altered. In fact, a type of gut bacteria responsible for preventing weight gain, diabetes, and disease and pathogen absorption decreased drastically.[25] Sugar is a primary culprit in weakening our gut bacteria and the gut-brain-hormone connection.

I recognize that eliminating the ultra-processed and high-sugar foods from your diet is a difficult process. However, I guarantee that the resulting longevity and improved mental and physical health are well worth it. If cutting out junk food from your pantry gave you 10 more healthy years of life, would you do it? I know my answer.

ALCOHOL EXPOSED

I hate to tell you, but it's time to break up with alcohol. While the inherent risks of alcohol are widely known, it continues to be a so-cially accepted vice for people to partake in during special occasions for celebration, during stressful situations as a coping tool, and ca-sually with dinner a few nights a week or even daily. However, the case against alcohol is a strong one. At age 60 or above, if you're a chronic drinker, you raise your risk of death by at least 20 percent.[26] If you don't drink alcohol regularly, keep doing what you're doing! For everyone else, this section serves to increase awareness of the real threat alcohol poses to longevity and to encourage you to cut it from your routine.

A groundbreaking study from 2022 compiled and analyzed data from over 36,000 adults and told us what we really needed to know about brain health and alcohol. The researchers found that one drink a day—just one—is enough to shrink the brain.[27] To think that having one glass of wine with dinner every night is enough to age the brain and to shrink it over time blows my mind, and I don't know how we didn't realize this sooner.

Alcohol has long been controversial in the medical and scientific communities. For years, countless doctors, me included, accepted research that found moderate alcohol consumption to be somewhat protective for brain and heart health. New studies totally negate that notion: If you drink nightly, the brain shrinks over time. We already know that alcohol is poison to our bodies and a gut bacteria killer, but this was the study that really made me rethink alcohol—let that fact sink in and inspire you to change your habits.

Quick Pause: Getting Real About Alcohol

Just one episode of binge drinking, a night out with friends, a wedding, a birthday party, can increase the risk of gut permeability. What does this mean? Alcohol causes bacteria to leak through the intestinal wall and pollute other parts of the body, which increases the amount of toxins in the blood and results in the body producing immune cells related to inflammation, cell destruction, and disease. Is that happy hour margarita pitcher worth it? Maybe not. I'm not here to bully you; believe me, I get it. But keep these ideas in mind next time alcohol is in the mix.

It should come as no surprise that limiting your alcohol consumption is a sure way to improve your health. Minimizing alcohol is especially important during the luteal phase of your cycle and in perimenopause when your hormone health is particularly vulnerable. Your gut acts as the control center for your hormone-brain connection, and when you're drinking alcohol, that control center becomes disoriented, and the accuracy and responsiveness of the gut become compromised. Maybe you've noticed that, after a night of drinking, you have more intense PMS or perimenopause symptoms. Alcohol prevents the gut from operating at its best, which then weakens the chain between your gut, your brain, and your hormones. Skipping alcohol will help in more ways than you might expect.

The effects of chronic alcohol consumption are exponential, meaning the more you drink, the more it shrinks your brain. If you're working toward improving your mental health and overall longevity, I urge you to give alcohol a break, maybe even permanently. For those of you who enjoy a drink with dinner or socially, that's okay, but I don't recommend having more than three or four drinks per week. Assessing your relationship with alcohol has never been more important than it is right now. We're learning more and more about how alcohol affects the brain each year, and it's projected that in the future we'll have even more data confirming the serious threat alcohol presents to our well-being.

Quick Pause: Alcohol Alternatives

Okay, so you're a social drinker and you don't want to miss out on the fun at the next girls' night out, wedding, birthday party, or whatever social event where alcohol is the norm. Maybe you've been pressured to drink at a social function when you'd rather not, or you're looking for ways to cut back on alcohol. Luckily for you, there are tons of great, nontoxic alternatives for alcohol you can turn to the next time you're out with friends or family and need some social lubricant.

For starters, you can walk into any bar or restaurant and order a mocktail—a drink that tastes great but lacks the poison. It will look like a cocktail, taste like a cocktail, and no one will be the wiser. "But isn't a mocktail just expensive juice?" Yes, yes, it is. However, it is still far better for you than the real deal. And it can be a great crutch when you're beginning to transition away from alcohol or lessen your alcohol intake.

Similarly, nonalcoholic beers and seltzers have become increasingly popular in that they give the illusion of cracking a cold one with friends but contain very little to no alcohol. For some, it's not so much the alcohol they enjoy but rather the social ritual of drinking. Nonalcoholic drinks are great alternatives when you don't want to drink but you're in an environment where drinking is the norm or expected.

A recent trend in the nonalcoholic beverage space are drinks containing CBD or adaptogens to help you relax without becoming intoxicated. For many people, winding down at the end of a stressful day with a glass of wine or cold pint is some much-needed relaxation. However, you can achieve these same calming effects through tasty nonalcoholic drinks designed to soothe without posing risks to your health.

It goes without saying that you can always ditch the facade of drinking and stick to water, soda, or whatever quenches your thirst. The bottom line is that, if your social circle treats you differently for opting for nonalcoholic beverages, they may not have your best interests at heart. If you need to be intoxicated to hang around certain people, they may not actually be your friend or someone you want to keep around. So much of breaking up with alcohol has to do with the circumstances in which we consume it and the people with whom we partake in it. No one criticizes a pregnant woman for abstaining from the champagne toast, and the same standard should be applied to anyone wanting to prioritize their health, pregnant or not. If you're wanting to change your relationship with alcohol, don't let anyone stand in the way of the healthy lifestyle you deserve.

WRAPPING UP NUTRITION

My patients often come to me because their doctors talk to them about medications but not supplements, and they feel lost when faced with managing symptoms of hormonal transition into perimeno-pause. A 47-year-old woman messaged me saying she talked to her doctor about perimenopause, and her doctor said to take vitamin D, lose weight, and eat a good diet. She said, "Before you, I didn't know what I should be doing. These things—perimenopause, hormones, and nutrition—were a mystery to me, but I've learned so much and feel more connected to my body, especially after taking magnesium."

This is not an isolated incident. I get messages on social media and from patients whose lives have changed within days of taking magnesium. However, the FDA does not have the same oversight on supplements as they do on medications, so many doctors feel more inclined to prescribe a drug than recommend a supplement to tackle nutritional deficiencies and perimenopause symptoms. Supplement companies are expected to follow guidelines, yet some don't, further decreasing the supplement industry's credibility in the eyes of medical professionals.

Further, it's the Wild West on the internet when it comes to nu-trition and supplementation. Women are targeted and bombarded with unreliable or misleading information about so-called miracle products, when what they really need is the knowledge of what is happening in the female body and how to optimize their hormone health. I'm not selling you a miracle—I'm giving you the tools to take your life and nutrition into your own hands.

I'll leave you with this thought: Your inputs become your outputs. This of course refers to the food, drinks, alcohol, sugar, and processed foods you take in. Your inputs are also your thoughts, habits, environ-ment, people you surround yourself with. Together, these manifest as your mood, energy levels, gut health, mental health, and physical health. These factors are the sum of your body and your life. What are you putting into your life? What are you putting into your mouth, into your brain?

If you're seeking a better output, create better inputs. That starts with nutrition.

CHAPTER 7

Supportive Mind-Gut Strategies

MOM, I SLIPPED IN THE bathroom and hit my chin. I thi—I think I broke something." My son broke his jaw on the eve of his sixteenth birthday, and his mouth had to be wired shut for a full month to heal. I still have PTSD from hearing his soft, broken voice on the other end of the line, and when I have bad dreams, the sounds of him screaming from pain still wake me up at night.

I had no way of knowing how much this horrific incident would impact me and my family for years to come. Little did I know that it would be Jaden's injury that spurred me on my journey to discover the power of nutrition and the mind-gut connection.

When Jaden broke his jaw, we were given very minimal nutrition advice except for an all-liquid diet. He'd spent the first month as a newly minted 16-year-old subsisting on Gatorade and juice—he couldn't even have smoothies because of the pulp! It didn't take long before his entire demeanor plummeted. My vibrant, happy-go-lucky boy was a shell of his normal self. Beyond not being able to eat real food, no one prepared him for the emotional-mental toll it takes on your body to *not* be able to speak or play sports for an extended period. Guidance on how to preserve his mental health was not part of his care plan; my son, just like anyone else would have, struggled with how to cope.

It was so frustrating seeing him suffer so much before my eyes, knowing that there wasn't anything I could do. We were following the advice prescribed by his doctor, yet it felt like there was something missing. Medicine was frustrating me left and right, and I began to dig deeper into the research behind using food to modulate the mind-gut connection. My son's broken jaw was just another glaring example to me of how modern medicine left so much on the table. My goal with this chapter, and this book, is to give you the life-enhancing tools you may have never received, especially when it comes to mind-body health.

Food is the most important tool you can use to unlock your potential and optimize your health, but there are several other strategies outside of your diet that you should use to your advantage to support that mind-gut connection. This chapter is all about understanding the inner workings of the mind-gut connection and the many supportive mind-gut strategies that will help you live better for longer.

Full disclosure: for a long time I didn't necessarily believe in the power of the mind over the body. I had never considered the benefits of mindset work to improve my or my patients' mental and physical well-being. We don't really talk much about the interconnectedness of the mind and body in medical school beyond a surface level, which is a shame.

It took me a lot of time, and I had to review a lot of research, to see the bigger picture: Our gut and brain are in constant communication with each other, which means that what we're consuming is what we're feeling, and what we're feeling is what we're consuming. This is seemingly obvious and overly simple, yet it's not something we're taught. As I've said, in medical school we are trained to assess the patient's symptoms to determine what is going on inside the body, prescribe treatment or medication to heal a specific issue, and monitor the patient's response to treatment. Rarely do we, as Western medical professionals, take a more holistic approach, which factors in a patient's environment, mental health, and lifestyle to determine if their condition is a result of many intertwined variables and could possibly be treated through unmedicated means.

Though discussions of nutrition and gut health are becoming more mainstream, the gut and brain relationship is still underestimated, or just plain misunderstood, by many. Let me put it this way: The gut and brain talk to each other constantly, and we cannot separate what we eat and do from how we think or feel. The mind-gut connection, also known as the brain-gut axis, is the facilitation of communication among biological networks such as neural pathways, the neuroendocrine and immune systems, and metabolic pathways. Our gut microbiome is known to influence our behaviors and can influence our chances of developing certain chronic illnesses or diseases.

Quick Pause: Inputs and Outputs

The brain and gut work together as the body's generals and they use the messengers by way of hormones and the nervous system to communicate. Cortisol and the emotions you feel are the messages being communicated between the brain and gut. To feel better, you need to change what you put into your gut and brain–this includes food, sunlight, stress, thoughts, media you consume, people you surround yourself with, and more. Think of these factors as your inputs, and how you feel and behave are your outputs.

This chapter is about understanding how the brain and gut are sending signals to the rest of the body. Speaking from personal experience, I've noticed so many benefits from changing my inputs, and I'm a complete believer in the power the mind-gut connection has over every aspect of our health. This understanding changed my life by helping me see my own gifts and develop lifestyle habits to live them out. When my inputs were really bad—I was not getting enough sleep, spending enough time in nature, or spending time with the people I love and friends who lift me up—I had a lot of hormonal, gut, and nervous system issues. It felt like there was an insurmountable roadblock of stress and fatigue that prevented me from living my best life.

I knew that I wasn't my best self and that I wasn't making the healthiest decisions for me—that's when it all fell into place. Using food and other supportive strategies to optimize my brain-gut connection was the ultimate game-changer. Your inputs create your outputs, and if you want to create better hormonal health, you need to change your inputs.

Do you remember that MODERN acronym from earlier? Surprise, it's back and better than before. MODERN is now HOT & MODERN:

H: Heat therapy
O: Own your morning
T: Build your tribe
M: Magnesium
O: Omega-3
D: Vitamin D
E: Exercise
R: Rest or sleep
N: Nutrition and Nature

You can think of the supportive mind-gut strategies in this chapter as a blueprint for bettering your inputs. We'll be diving into strategies related to your attitude, stress resilience, sleep, sunlight, work-life balance, and community. Supportive strategies for optimizing your mind-gut connection differ from self-care in that the strategies we'll go over in this chapter are habits you should practice over time. For example, having ample sleep, getting sufficient sunlight, and having a strong support system is not self-care—these elements are essential for life. If splurging on a ten-dollar iced coffee, taking a bubble bath, getting a facial, having a movie marathon, or any other self-care indulgence makes you happy, then absolutely keep doing those things! You should be aware, however, that the positive emotions you experience from treating yourself do not equate to the long-term benefits from changing your inputs and developing practical habits for longevity and optimized brain, gut, and hormone health.

Changing your inputs means prioritizing your mental health, being intentional about the people you spend time with and media you consume, listening to your body, and understanding how resilience improves health outcomes. Let's dive in.

ATTITUDE

The first mind-gut supportive strategy is centered on attitude. I talked about the mind-body connection earlier, and it's important to understand how our attitude impacts mental and physical health. The negative thoughts you may have about yourself or the cynical lens through which you may look at the world are examples of harmful mental inputs within your control that negatively influence the mind-gut connection.

Here is a vulnerable story that I'm not proud of but feel obligated to share. Recently, as I started to have a larger following on social media, I received an opportunity to partner with a brand that I admired. It's a prominent brand name that many people would know, and I couldn't be more excited to work with them.

When I got there to film the content, they started briefing me on their company and their ideal customer. They talked about their brand ethos and how they were really targeting the woman in her twenties. I thought about how my friends and I really loved the brand, but we were clearly outside the age range of their target audience. During the briefing, I started to feel embarrassed to even be a part of this opportunity because of my age. I wondered, "Do they even know how old I am?"

I became so self-conscious that I couldn't shake negative thoughts about my age for the whole day. I became hyperaware that a lot of the people in the room were at least 10 if not 20 years younger than me. I spent the entire experience, something I was initially so excited about, second-guessing my worth and wishing I had started doing social media when I was younger (between medical school, becoming a mother, and working as a doctor . . . yeah, there was totally time to take on social media, too, right?). When I was looking at the content a few weeks later, I was instantly transported back to that moment and the torrent of harmful thoughts and emotions I experienced during the shoot.

Although I'm embracing perimenopause and my journey along the hormonal continuum, I recognized in that specific instance my insecurities around aging, and the aging process derailed my enthusiasm for a project I was super passionate about. Looking back, I wish I had been more aware of my thoughts and tried harder to re-center myself in the moment. This experience showed me just how powerful a negative attitude can be, how much it can take something that's supposed to fulfill me and turn it into something sour and miserable.

I share this story as a reminder that life isn't always how it may seem on social media. I have my bad days just like everyone else, and I have days where I don't feel like I'm enough—even though I know

I am. I have a family that I love with all my heart, and I'm fantastic at my multifaceted job as a doctor and health advocate. We all have our moments where we let negativity get the best of us, and that's okay. What's important, though, is that we are equipped with strategies to pull ourselves out of dark places, overcome our mind, and shift our attitude.

You can change your inputs by refocusing your mindset and energy to center yourself. I know it's difficult, but try to be kinder to yourself and focus on the love around you, your success and well-being, and that of loved ones. Despite how it may feel some days, you *do* have power over your brain, and you can acknowledge your negative thoughts or stress and let them go.

Quick Pause: We Are What's in Our Gut

Did you know that your gut bacteria have the power to change your mental state and even influence your personality? A recent study from the University of Oxford analyzed the microbiome-gut-brain axis of 655 participants and found that gut microbiome composition and diversity are in fact linked to personality traits.[1] This study yielded several poignant findings, but the takeaways that stood out most were:

1. People with larger social circles and people who travel frequently have more diverse microbial communities.
2. People with low diversity in their gut microbiome display higher levels of stress and anxiety.
3. People who eat foods high in probiotics and prebiotics have significantly lower levels of stress and anxiety, and they are less likely to suffer from mental illness.

Another study examined the link between gut bacteria and mental illnesses, specifically schizophrenia.[2] The researchers took gut bacteria samples from patients who had schizophrenia and patients who did not have schizophrenia, and they gave these samples to mice that had no bacteria at all. The mice containing these new gut bacteria were observed together as a group. The researchers were able to tell which mice had gotten the schizophrenic patients' gut bacteria just from their behavior. They did nothing to the mice's brains, yet the brains of the mice changed drastically due to the gut bacteria they received.

Whether or not it's obvious, your attitude is a core input that influences all aspects of health. If you're someone who is prone to mood swings or you can't remember the last time you smiled, this is for you. While we may not be in total control of our mental health, we can be in control of the way we treat others and ourselves. Maybe the barista made you the wrong drink. Rather than jump to anger or annoyance, step back from your emotions (while acknowledging them), and proceed with kindness and understanding. Or maybe you fumbled an important meeting at work and mentally berated yourself for the rest of the day. Recognize the intense emotions you're experiencing and allow yourself to move past them, focusing on the next thing. In other words, don't sweat the small stuff.

Emotions have the capacity to reveal greater truths about us. Take anger, for example. When we are angry about something, it's because a boundary has been crossed, even if we didn't realize that boundary was there. Emotions like jealousy, fear, or shame may highlight parts of ourselves that need acceptance or our desire to change. As women, we're simultaneously seen as overly emotional and told to suppress what we feel. This leads to barriers in expressing ourselves and bottling up what we truly feel until our emotions inevitably boil over after being pushed down for so long. Let me just say that your emotions are valid. You have every right to feel what you feel. Don't suppress emotions, but do pay attention to what your emotions might be telling you. Emotions can be your best teacher.

Acknowledging the overwhelming thoughts or emotions then letting them go is a fundamental aspect of meditation. While it may not be for everyone, many people experience mind-calming benefits from meditation, and it's worth giving a try if you have trouble with your mood. You could also try journaling, which is a great outlet for expressing what you're feeling. When you're able to recognize harmful shifts in your attitude and correct course, you're setting yourself up for greater mental stability and a stronger mind-gut connection.

I have an exercise I like to do with my family, especially after super rough days, called "Rose, Thorn, and Rosebud." You may have heard of this. It's simple, takes only a few minutes, and gives everyone an opportunity to speak about their day and decompress. I do this with my family, but you can do this with your partner, a friend, or even on your own in a journal. Your "rose" is something positive from the day—it can be something as small as the lunch you had or something big like getting a promotion. The "thorn" is something negative from your day—an opportunity to vent and have others hear your frustrations rather than hold on to them. And the "rosebud" is supposed to be something you are looking forward to or a goal. Another common iteration of this exercise is to talk about a "peak" and "pit" from the day, but I personally like the addition of the rosebud, which ensures that the conversation always ends on a hopeful note.

For example, today my rose was that I went on a beautiful morning hike and took in the stunning scenery to calm my mind before starting the workday. My thorn was that I hit every red light on the way to a meeting and ended up being 5 minutes late (the horror!). My rosebud was that I'm super excited about a new study I read today and want to brainstorm ideas of how to communicate this new information to my followers. See, it's not so hard. By verbalizing these thoughts to my family, I can feel myself letting go of the anxiety and self-loathing I felt earlier in the day when I was late. I'm also able to speak my intentions surrounding new social media content and shelve that idea for the next day.

Why is something like this important? I know that it's a little silly, but it provides an outlet for me to talk through my day, my triumphs, frustrations, and worries, instead of going to bed and letting my mind run free. Like so many others, I struggle with turning off my rampant thoughts that keep me up into the night. This exercise (in combination with other sleep optimization strategies I'll get to shortly) lessens the mental load I bring to my pillow. It's also another way for me to connect with my family. I know firsthand the chaos that is being a mother to teenagers, and during it all, it's important for me to check in with my kids to see how they're *really* feeling. The conversations that stem (ha) from the rose-thorn-rosebud exercise go beyond surface level and allow us to be vulnerable with one another. This means more effective communication, deeper emotional connection, and, ultimately, growth. I encourage you to give this simple exercise a try; you may be surprised by how much breaking down your day into these three categories can reshape your attitude into one of hope for what is yet to come.

Quick Pause: Bonus Exercise

Grab a piece of paper and something to write with. I prefer you not do this one in the notes app on your phone–writing it down takes more time and will let you sit with your thoughts more closely.

Okay, now write down five things you like about yourself. Really. That's it! For some of you, this may sound super easy, while for others this could be a struggle. I want you to think about five qualities that you love about yourself and the value that you bring.

Here's my list:

1. I love my unquenchable thirst for knowledge and how it causes me to always dig deeper and challenge my beliefs.
2. I am a good mother, and I've raised two strong, kindhearted children.
3. I love my job, and I am grateful every day that I get to help others.
4. I'm a dependable friend, and I like that I prioritize being there for them as much as they are there for me.
5. I like that I carve out time to go outside almost every day to connect with nature, exercise, and quiet my brain.

My list takes a look at the big picture of my life and what I appreciate about myself, but you can also write about smaller things like "I love my new haircut," "I think I handled a difficult situation at work very professionally, and I'm proud of that," or "I put fifty dollars into my vacation fund today because when I set a goal, I stick to it." No matter the approach you take to making your list, the aim is to practice uninhibited self-love.

We can be our own worst enemy, and this journal exercise will help you dig your thoughts out of a pit of unchecked self-loathing, doubt, and resentment. When you're done, stick it on the bathroom mirror or refrigerator if you feel so inclined. You are worthy, you are valid, and you have so much to offer the world. Sometimes we just need a little reminder.

MIND-BODY EMOTIONAL STRESS

Let's pivot slightly and talk about stress, which is a direct influence on our attitude and, really, every aspect of mental health. Stress is what we experience when there is an imbalance between the demands of what's happening in our lives and our ability to respond to those demands. Our perceptions of the stressors in our lives cause various physiological and behavioral responses that manifest in ways according to the level of threat we interpret the stressor to have. We all experience stress to different degrees, and it is, for better or worse, an inherent part of the human condition.

Quick Pause: Stress and Perimenopause

You're more sensitive to stress. And I don't mean you, the reader, are more sensitive to stress than I am—what I mean is, biologically, you and I are more sensitive to stress during these years of perimenopause and menopause than we have ever been, and we need our sleep as much as possible.

Stress is known to be linked to increased risk of depression, cardiovascular disease, dementia, Alzheimer's, and accelerated aging. For women in perimenopause, high levels of stress can cause issues with sleep, mood disorders, and even worsen symptoms like hot flashes.

We all have a lot of stress in our lives, whether emotional stress; stress from work, family, or relationships; financial stress; or just a general sense of being stressed out that we can't seem to shake. The goal is to decrease all of that, but there also should be a special focus on the stress load you're exerting on your body. I'm talking about the physical stress your body endures daily as you move along the hormonal continuum.

If you're staying up late and skimping on sleep, having a ton of caffeine, doing multiple high-intensity workouts per week, doing a really long fast, and then expecting your body to recover from all of these stressors at once, you are sorely mistaken. Your body does not react well to high levels of stress during perimenopause, and it gets more and more difficult for the body to cope with stress as we age.

For the health of your hormones and the mind-gut connection, think about the various stress-inducing variables in your life that are within your control. In a culture where we are encouraged to do more and more, I'm asking you how you can do less. Can you try going to bed 30 minutes or even an hour earlier? Is the frequency of your workouts having a detrimental impact on your body's ability to recover—would you benefit more from a gentle walk in nature rather than another intense class this week? What about signing up for a grocery-delivery service or meal prepping to make your load easier? Can you cut back on your caffeine intake? These questions can help you identify areas where you can lessen the stress on your mind and body.

I don't expect stress management to be as simple as a few minutes of self-reflection; in fact, it took me years to dial back my lifestyle habits to where they are now, and I still experience high levels of stress fairly often. However, the work I have done, and continue to do, to manage my stress over time is going to significantly benefit my postmenopausal self when I arrive at that stage in life. It's important to remember that the aging process has already started (the clock doesn't start ticking when you turn 30; it starts ticking at birth), but you have the capacity to positively influence the trajectory of your health into old age. Effective stress management is crucial for healthy aging.

A recent meta-analysis on the efficacy of stress management methods for reducing cortisol levels found the category of stress interventions described as "mindfulness" to be the most effective, followed by "meditation" as the second most effective intervention category across more than fifty studies.[3] In healthy adults, mind work is shown to be very effective in helping to mitigate the negative effects associated with high stress. The mind is powerful and can be harnessed for both harm and health, depending on how we frame it. If we devote our energy to focusing on our worries and things beyond our control, our mind and body will suffer. However, if we learn to control our response to stressors, mental-emotional stress will take less of a physical toll on the body.

Think about the exercises you do. Think about the people you spend time with. Think about your activities on a typical day. The goal is to feel rejuvenated, not depleted, on a regular basis. I can guarantee the lifestyle that worked for you in your twenties is not going to work for you now. You will need to make changes to work toward decreasing both your physical and mental stressors. Stress takes a toll on your body, and it's never too late to work on lessening that load.

Once you've worked on diet, sleep, and the areas of your life that contribute the most to your stress load, give yourself an outlet you can consistently utilize to cool down, de-stress, and center yourself. A lot of people find meditation before bed to be super helpful in winding down from the day and priming the mind for a good night's sleep. Other stress-relief outlets to consider are restorative yoga, walking, breathing exercises, music, reading, or any activity that allows you to turn down the noise in your head and come out of it feeling lighter.

Quick Pause: Take a Breath

Let's walk through a quick five-minute breathing exercise you can do anywhere to center yourself when you're feeling overwhelmed with the various stressors life throws your way.

Find a quiet place for yourself and get comfortable. You can do this exercise standing, sitting, lying down, in a simple yoga pose, or in any position you prefer. If you're standing, place your feet shoulder-width apart with your arms at your sides. If you're lying down, your can straighten your legs or bend your knees, feet flat on the floor, with your arms away from your sides, palms facing upward. If you're sitting, place your hands either in your lap or on the arms of the chair, feet flat on the ground.

Now breathe. To focus on your breath, you can close your eyes once you begin the exercise. Breathe deeply, but don't push yourself to breathe deeper than what feels natural. Breathe in through your nose, out through your mouth. You can visualize the breath going from deep within your belly, up and out through your mouth, and into the world. Let these breaths you release represent the thoughts and worries contributing to your stress.

Breathe in. Breathe out–let it go. Try counting to five on the inhale and exhale, but don't worry if you can't make it to five. The goal here is to get 5 minutes of deep breathing, no distractions. I encourage you to take a few minutes to try this exercise and think about how your body feels afterward. What do you notice? Were you clenching your jaw all day without even noticing? Did you drop your shoulders? Notice these changes and observe the link between your mind and body, the toll stress takes both mentally and physically.

Spend some time analyzing the stressors you face in your life. Which stressors are within your control, and which ones are beyond your reach? What are some small changes you can make today that will minimize the effects of those stressors? How are your diet and sleep? Finally, what are some stress-relief tactics you can incorporate into your routine to set yourself up for a good night of restful sleep? Knowing how to manage your stress level will help decrease that sense of fight or flight your brain sends to the rest of the body, making it easier to strengthen the mind-gut connection.

MINDSET

Here is the secret health weapon for women we don't talk about enough: mindset. How do we manage our minds in such a chaotic world? Twenty years ago, when I was in India shopping for my wedding, my mom was seated next to a gentleman named Ram in one of the shops. My mom is not the one you want to be seated next to if you don't want to converse at all. She will smile, offer to share her snacks, and ask where you are going. Ram was an enthusiastic elderly man in his seventies with a graying mustache, and he was excited to let her know that this was perhaps the most important trip of his life.

"Why is that?" my mom inquired. He told her his family had a sari store in south India and there was a buyer who wanted to make the biggest purchase in his business's 35-year history, but they would decide tonight. "Oh, wow! You must be nervous," my mom said. "I wouldn't be able to sleep!"

"Well," he said, "I've had ways for dealing with uncertainty all my life. It's spirituality. I believe there is a higher power, and whenever I get a large deal, I donate a substantial portion of it to charity and the temple as tribute." He explained to my mom that if the deal went through, half of the money would be donated in honor of the spiritual creator who made it possible.

They continued talking, and she asked him more about his spiritual beliefs in business and otherwise. He said that having this belief had protected him from worry, stress, and feelings of anger or irritability. He felt that his beliefs had made him a better father, husband, and business owner. "I owe my sanity to spirituality," he told her.

My mom was so taken by his passion and excitedly told us the story as we walked through Bengaluru airport. Ram's story left quite an impression on me at the time because I was studying medicine, only a few months out from graduation. I started to think about the biological ways in which spirituality works to calm the nervous system. I was less concerned about how real it was or the spiritual figures he believed in; rather, I was interested in how it could help our brain.

I forgot about Ram's story until I started my wellness business and perimenopause symptoms knocked on my door. As I moved through partnership deals and sponsors, I started to feel uncertainty and have exaggerated sleep problems, and I desperately needed a way to channel my anxiety of the unknown. I needed to take all the uncertainty I was feeling and turn it into something positive.

That's where mindset comes in. Mindset is simply the unique lens through which we view the world, and we have the power to shape it. It's your expectations, assumptions, and projections of yourself and the world around you. Your mindset is how you take in your surroundings and adapt.

Quick Pause: Fixed vs. Growth Mindset

Dr. Carol Dweck, whom you may already know, is a prolific psychologist known for her work in the areas of motivation and mindset. She introduced the ideas of "fixed" and "growth" mindsets to describe the diverse ways people approach moving through life.[4]

A *fixed mindset* applies to someone who believes their abilities, intelligence, and development are static, that they cannot be drastically changed or influenced over time. A *growth mindset* applies to those who notice potential within themselves to constantly improve in all areas of life. Now, it may sound like I'm making fixed mindsets out to be a terrible thing, but they aren't. There are benefits to having a fixed mindset about some facets of life; for example, a fixed belief in one's love for their friends and family, or a fixed belief in one's role in their community. A fixed mindset can reinforce one's sense of confidence but, when applied to every aspect of life, can hinder positive development necessary for personal growth.

Having a growth mindset means that you seek opportunities that challenge you, you take mistakes as moments for learning, and you recognize qualities about yourself that can be improved upon. While this type of mindset is largely constructive, when taken too far it can lead to self-doubt, perfectionism, and overthinking. I don't share these concepts with you in hopes that you pick one or the other, but rather that you start to recognize the types of mindsets you carry through your life. Do you want to be someone who continues to learn new skills as they age? Are you open to different perspectives and learning from others? What is your role in different relationships in your life, with friends, family, and your community? What about your life fulfills you most? What do you want to do more of? These are some questions worth considering to identify when your mindset is fixed and when you have a growth mindset.

Unlike our genes, mindset is a characteristic about ourselves that we can control and change over and over throughout our life. The entire field of cognitive therapy is rooted in the belief that anyone can learn to develop a healthier way of thinking. We can all learn to notice when our thoughts are bringing us down and redirect them to more neutral and positive outlooks for the benefit of the brain and our well-being. Similarly, we can choose how we react to outside triggers. Mel Robbins talks about this notion at length in her book *The Let Them Theory*; the nexus of her ideology is that when someone is being rude or annoying, say to yourself, "Let them," and free yourself from whatever it is they may be thinking or feeling about you.[5] This style of mindset is something we can all embody to work on our stress management and learn not to sweat the small stuff. We will inevitably be subject to several things that frustrate us every single day, and it's up to us how we respond.

Given that we are more prone to stress and its negative physical side effects as we go through perimenopause, having a powerful mindset is our secret weapon for optimized hormonal transition and aging. Mindset work is the most valuable form of self-care you can practice. When you're in control of you—your thoughts, your reactions, your emotions—you have the power to transcend whatever challenge you may be facing. You got this (but only if you think so)!

SLEEP

I've spoken about how crucial it is to have healthy sleep habits during perimenopause and for optimizing hormone, brain, and gut health, but let's go a little deeper into how sleep fits in as a supportive strategy for optimizing the mind-gut connection. The circadian rhythm is your body's best friend, compass, and clock. It's what governs your sleep, hunger, and energy to help maximize your available resources.

Sleep, along with nutrition, is the input with the greatest impact on the mind-gut connection and, really, any process of the body. The circadian rhythm is our own personal clock that regulates the sleep-wake cycle and affects hunger, eating habits, and digestion. Resetting the circadian rhythm can be approached in many ways. For example, morning sunlight provides you with energy for the day, and sticking to regular mealtimes will allow digestion and metabolism to influence feelings of sleepiness or wakefulness. Prioritizing stress management balances a part of our body that is closely related to the circadian rhythm.

Many of us have unintentionally put sleep on the back burner due to the demands of our busy lives. Sleep affects the part of the brain that processes our inhibition, and without it, we are much more likely to make unhealthy choices and decisions. A good night's rest is proven to be a trusty, natural appetite suppressant and supports our ability to think, reason, react, and respond. Adequate sleep normalizes hormone levels and gives the body the chance to create order among them. Sleep is so incredibly important.

A lot of women suffer from changes in their quality of sleep during perimenopause whether it's the inability to fall asleep, hot flashes, night sweats, nighttime awakenings, and more. A lot of us suffer from cortisol awakenings that typically happen between 2 and 4 a.m. You're in a light sleep when suddenly you get this cortisol bump in the middle of the night, and it wakes you up, making it difficult to fall back to sleep. Knowing how to set yourself up for a good night of sleep is important in preventing these cortisol spikes in the middle of the night.

My hope is that you become sleep obsessed like I am. If you're someone who suffers with sleep issues during perimenopause, you're going to have to work hard to get your circadian rhythm back on track. You can consider trying products like blackout curtains or wearing an eye mask at night to get a superior sleep. Before going to bed, maybe take a little bit of melatonin, magnesium, chamomile, L-theanine, or valerian root. You generally need to drop your temperature by 1 degree Fahrenheit to be able to fall asleep, so make sure your bedroom is cool and use blankets that won't be too warm. You should be wary of drinking caffeine in the afternoon, and refrain from having alcohol before bed, which really does disturb circadian rhythms and your ability to sleep through the night.

One of the most important things I tell women in perimenopause is that you don't have to get a full 8 hours of sleep every single night. It's just not feasible for so many of us. My recommendation is to aim for at least 3 nights of great, restful sleep per week. If you're getting more than four nights of restorative sleep per week, you're doing a fantastic job!

Quick Pause: 3, 2, 1 . . . Sleep!

Having trouble falling asleep? Try the 10-3,2,1,0 method:

Ten hours before you go to sleep, no caffeine. For many of us, this means having our last cup of coffee, or whatever your preferred source of caffeine, by around noon. Drinking caffeine throughout the day makes it harder to calm the mind and fall asleep. Though decaf isn't wholly caffeine-free, try switching out your afternoon or evening caffeinated beverage with decaf for better sleep at night.

Three hours before bed, you should not be eating anything. I understand this can be challenging at times. Who doesn't love a midnight snack? Well, our mind and gut certainly don't. If you eat dinner at 6 or 7 p.m., you should have about 3 hours without food before bed. Eating right before going to bed is bad for digestion and bad for your sleep, which means that little nighttime snack isn't worth the negative impacts it will have later on. Now, I understand that many people have demanding work schedules that make this difficult. If it takes you an hour to commute home; an hour to get groceries, go to the gym, or spend time with family; an hour to make a meal, then it's likely you don't have 3 hours to wait before going to bed. I totally get it. Try as much as you can to limit eating before bed, but if you slip from time to time, it isn't the end of the world. Perhaps there are easy shifts you can make to your routine—like bringing dinner with you to work to have on the commute home or ending your workday a bit earlier—so that you can eat earlier and then sleep better.

Two hours of strictly no work before bed. This means no work-related phone calls, no checking your email, no working on that last-minute assignment within 2 hours of bedtime. This also applies to any other task or form of media that serves as a stressor in your life, such as watching the news in bed, speaking on the phone with a family member who you maybe don't want to talk to, checking your credit card statement, or analyzing your schedule for the week and realizing there aren't enough hours in the day. The aim here is to limit exposure to high-stress triggers and to spend the 2 hours before bed relaxing and preparing our mind and body for sleep. Focus on cutting out work and blue lights at least 2 hours before bedtime so that, when it's time to crawl into bed, your mind is calm enough to shut off for the night.

One hour before bed, turn off all your devices. That includes putting away your phone—no scrolling through social media, watching YouTube or Netflix, or online shopping within an hour of falling asleep. For a lot of us, this is the hardest thing to do. Even if it's only 30 minutes, cutting out screen time before bed is going to improve your quality of sleep. There are apps that limit your screen time for you, so if you try to use social media outside of the window you set for yourself, you won't be able to do so. Part of getting better sleep is working on improving our relationship with our phones and social media. Adolescents are particularly susceptible to a technology addiction, but people of all ages are becoming increasingly glued to their devices, which has serious negative effects on physical, psychological, and social health.[6] Addiction to our phones can actually cause depression. That's powerful stuff. You don't need to break up with your phone, but limiting your screen time can only serve to benefit your mental health and promote better sleep.

Zero is the number of times you should be hitting snooze in the morning. Why? When you hit snooze and fall back asleep, you get back into deep REM and non-REM sleep. By hitting snooze, you start a new sleep cycle, which is 45 minutes. When the alarm goes off again, you're even groggier than the first time because you woke in the middle of two incomplete sleep cycles, making it more difficult to start your day. Strive to wake up as soon as your alarm goes off. Believe me, I hate waking up to an alarm. I just want to keep hitting snooze over and over. To avoid starting my morning with a thunderous alarm in my ear, I try to time my bedtime so that I'm not sleeping past my alarm. When I practice good sleep hygiene and get to bed early enough, I'm able to wake up before my alarm. Now I set an alarm just in case of emergencies.

If you're someone who frequently wakes up between 2 and 4 in the morning, this is a sign that your stress levels are out of control. The good news is that you can get control of these cortisol-fueled wakeups once you learn how to wind down from the day. For example, if I disconnect from work about 2 hours before bed, I'm able to sleep through the night much better than if I'm staying up responding to emails until my eyes close for the night. Give the 10–3,2,1,0 method a try and see if it helps you get to sleep quicker and stay asleep through the night.

For my night owls, let this be your wakeup call (full pun intended). A 2024 study from Stanford University analyzed more than seventy thousand adults and found that people who went to bed and woke up earlier had better mental health.[7] Period. The researchers recommended going to bed before 10 p.m. for healthy aging and brain health protection as we get older. Further, a separate study identified a link between gut microbiome diversity and quality of sleep.[8] People with more diverse gut microbiomes got longer, more restful sleep with less instances of waking in the middle of the night. Food and sleep are your most powerful tools for taking control of your health and ensuring that the best years of your life are ahead of you.

SUNLIGHT

Sunlight is another valuable tool to have in your mind-gut toolbox. Getting adequate light into your eyes, even on a cloudy day, is a vital way to optimize your brain-gut-hormone connection. Adequate exposure to sunlight is known to regulate the circadian rhythm and sleep patterns and increase quality of sleep. Sunlight also promotes vitamin D production; boosts serotonin, productivity, energy, and mood; and also regulates melatonin. Plants need sunlight to survive, and so do we.

Sunlight is beneficial for us any time of day, but the morning is when it's most vital. When you get sunshine within an hour of waking, it triggers a neural circuit responsible for the release of cortisol and melatonin, which greatly impact our sleep. While any sunlight is going to greatly benefit your circadian rhythm, try to get outdoors and go for a walk. Our windows filter some of the ultraviolet light that promotes the regulation of our body's internal clock, as do sunglasses. Don't take this to mean you need to stare into the sun to sleep better at night, because that isn't the case; but do your best to get outside and enjoy the sunshine (or cloudy skies) before getting your day started.

Getting sunlight into your eyes in the morning resets your circadian rhythm, your body's clock, and it redefines what time it is to your brain and your body by telling your hormones, "Okay, it's time to fire." It also tells your GI tract that it's time to turn on. When you regularly get natural light in the morning, you're able to recalibrate these clocks all around your body and especially that master clock in your brain. By doing so, you will feel better. When your brain and body clocks are misaligned, it's like feeling perpetually jet-lagged.

Spending too much time in the dark, not getting enough sunlight in the daytime, or getting a lot of bright blue light at night causes that jet-lagged sense of exhaustion that can affect your mood and productivity and influence a host of health concerns with disrupted circadian rhythm. Sunsets are known to be beneficial as well; soft evening light can help signal to the brain that the day is coming to an end, thus triggering the release of adequate melatonin for sleep.

Quick Pause: Mother Nature

This all sounds so obvious, yet we often forget the undisputable link between humans and the natural world. Our increasingly digital world is not in fact natural, and we must make conscious efforts each day to get outside and reconnect with nature. Living a life with screens always less than a foot away from our eyes will have both mental and physical consequences later. Do what you can now to establish healthier relationships with blue-light devices and make sunshine a priority. As a bonus, sunlight is free and accessible to all!

We know that getting outdoors has tremendous benefits for nearly every aspect of our health; however, what's more urgent is the detrimental effects of *not* going outside. *The Nature Fix* by Florence Williams talks about this idea in depth, but what you need to know is that not getting outside can trigger and worsen depression, anxiety, and other mental disorders, especially in children.[9]

There were several studies conducted across the world that found spending time outside improves cognitive function, making us more creative, better problem solvers, more critical thinkers, and more attentive.[10,11] The more time you spend outdoors, the more your brain can rest and recharge, which is yet another benefit of getting sunshine shortly after waking up.

A 2010 study from Japan observed the physiological effects of *shinrin-yoku,* or "forest bathing," simply spending time in nature.[12] The researchers collected data from 280 participants in twenty-four forests across Japan with the aim of understanding our biological response to natural surroundings as opposed to city settings. What they found was that the participants engaging with forest environments exhibited lowered cortisol levels, pulse rate, blood pressure, and sympathetic nerve activity (think of this as the part of your brain in charge of fight or flight) with increased parasympathetic nerve activity compared to participants immersed in city environments. Parasympathetic nerve activity refers to the components of the nervous system that are in charge of conserving energy and regulating digestion, your "rest and digest" part of the nervous system. In simple terms, the participants in the forest environments were calmer, more at rest, than the participants in the city setting. While this may seem overly simplistic–"Duh, Dr. Shah, I'm obviously more at peace sitting by a lake than in rush hour traffic"–this study highlights the significance of the relationship between the natural world and human health as well as the role and merit of nature in preventative medicine. Ultimately, nature is medicine; it makes us feel better and literally improves our health through the simple act of being in the presence of our natural world, which is something screens can't replicate.

Having the time to get outdoors is a luxury many of us cannot afford among the many demanding aspects of our lives. However, get outside whenever you can as much as you can. Perhaps you can go for a walk with your family after dinner, take your lunch break outside when the weather is nice, go on a hike or visit a park at least once per week, or have your morning coffee out on the porch. There is no one-size-fits-all protocol for how we should be interacting with Mother Nature, but the bottom line is that we need to spend more time connecting with nature for the sake of our health.

I cannot stress this enough: Having regular access to sunlight or a sunlamp (like the ones some people in northern parts of the world use in winter when sunlight is scarce) is crucial. Don't under-estimate a resource as fundamental as sunlight! Getting sunlight in the morning is optimal. But getting it any time of the day is helpful in resetting your circadian rhythm and sleep cycle. I'm always telling everyone to get sunlight in the morning, preferably while going for a walk outside. We know that spending time in nature, even if it's just a green space in the city, has a tremendous impact on our mental and physical well-being. Spending time outside, getting light into your eyes, is linked to better sleep, lower blood pressure, and lower risk of developing chronic diseases.

A recent study published in *Cell Metabolism* identified a link be-tween gut bacteria and the body's response to stress.[13] Researchers noted that the depletion of gut bacteria has the capacity to impair the body's stress response in a circadian rhythm dependent manner. What this means is that when you get sufficient sunlight and time in nature, you can help your gut bacteria regulate hormones. Poor gut health impacts hormone health in significant ways, so by getting outside for at least an hour a day, you can strengthen your circadian rhythm and protect the gut-brain axis.

The benefits sunlight has in terms of the circadian rhythm, sleep, vitamin D, and mental health simultaneously contribute to strength-ening the mind-gut connection. Sunlight is a vital input every per-son needs, but especially those looking to optimize their hormone health and longevity.

COMMUNITY

We are who we surround ourselves with, quite literally. There's ev-idence that, yes, the people we surround ourselves with influence changes in the gut microbiome. In the study from University of Ox-ford that I introduced earlier, people with larger social circles are known to have more diverse gut bacteria, which shows that how we socialize is linked to our gut health, which, as we know, is linked to everything else in the body.

Beyond the gut health benefits from being a social butterfly, human connection can lower your risk of death by 50 percent. What does that even mean? As we get older, it's essential that we have a strong supportive network and outlets for socializing. We know that adolescents and teens thrive in their mental health when they have more social connections, and this trend continues into adulthood. We also know that risk of disease and struggles with mental health go down significantly when you have fulfilling social connections. A recent study found that people between the ages of 40 and 59 experience the most negative effects associated with a lack of belonging within their community, more than any other age group.[14] Community is a crucial aspect of health that becomes even more important as we age. For women in particular, the "Female Friendship Effect" (FFE) is my term for the unique benefits women get from being with each other. FFE increases oxytocin, opioids, our immune system, and reduces cortisol!

It's not about having more connections; rather, it's about having meaningful connections. The quality of your relationships plays a pivotal role in your physical health and longevity.

As you get older, it's also important that you have a sense of community, people in your day-to-day who you maybe don't have strong connections with but who can check in when they sense something is off. For example, do you live in a neighborhood where people notice if you haven't been out in a few days? Are you part of an exercise class or some other group where people will note your absence? Are you a regular at a coffee shop or local business where the employees would wonder if you didn't pop in for a few weeks? When we feel as though we are an active member of a community, we have a greater sense of purpose and feel more valued. Having a strong community outside of the family unit or friend group also means we have a greater network to rely on when we need it most.

If you're someone with social anxiety or you struggle with forging connections with others, know that you're not alone. I understand that socializing does not come so easily to many of us. However, I will say that being part of a community and building connections in person are vital to our health as humans. Some people think that online connection is enough, but it isn't. You need in-person contact with others to improve your health and longevity.

THE BOTTOM LINE

The best way to optimize the brain-gut connection is first and foremost through food. Once you master your nutrition, slowly implement these strategies one after the other until they become habits.

Everybody's journey through the hormonal continuum is different, and the changes our bodies go through are different for every woman. We all have unique struggles with health, and how we address those issues is unique to our needs and lifestyle. At the root of it, every woman in perimenopause needs sunlight, sleep, social connection, and outlets for stress. Use the strategies in this chapter to address those facets of the mind-gut connection on your own terms.

CHAPTER 8

Movement and Exercise

W E'VE ALL HEARD THE ADAGE that motion is lotion, which is true. It's also somewhat of a happy pill. Wouldn't you know that exercise can be as effective as antidepressants? A *JAMA* meta-analysis from 2024 involving more than 14,100 participants found that exercise, such as walking, jogging, yoga, and strength training, may help treat depression.[1] It turns out that working out does more than just burn calories, but you already knew that.

With the right type of exercise, you can gain control of your hormones, neurotransmitters, and other bodily chemicals. Exercise, especially in nature, drastically improves mood and mental health. It calms the brain and may bring relief to those who feel drawn to food when met with difficult emotions. When we get moving, three key neurotransmitters are activated and spur significant changes in the brain: (1) serotonin, (2) dopamine, and (3) gamma-aminobutyric acid (GABA).

Quick Pause: Neurotransmitter Refresher

Serotonin is a natural chemical in the body that transports messages between cells in the brain and throughout the rest of the body. It is integral to our mood, sleeping habits, digestion, stress resilience, bone health, and more.

Like serotonin, dopamine is a chemical messenger communicating within the brain and throughout the body, but

---

it also acts as a hormone. It's known as the "feel-good hormone" because it's intricately linked to our evolutionary reward system, meaning that our brains are programmed to make us behave certain ways and do certain things that then release dopamine.

Finally, gamma-aminobutyric acid (GABA) is another chemical messenger in the brain that blocks specific signals in the central nervous systems (CNS) to slow down the brain. GABA is known for producing a calming effect and lowers the activity of cells in the brain and nervous system. Its calming effect can prevent the use of overindulging and overeating as coping mechanisms.

Why should you exercise? Because it will make you feel good. Seriously. Maybe not in the immediate moment of doing a push-up, going for a jog, or participating in a hot yoga class, but I promise the aftermath of the suffering we may endure during exercise is bliss. By working out, your brain will release these vital neurotransmitters and ultimately improve the hypothalamus-pituitary-adrenal axis, boost your mood, support your mental health, and even curb hunger and cravings. Regular physical activity is known to help with various psychiatric disorders, sleep issues, anxiety, and even addiction.[2] Exercise has the capacity to improve so many different aspects of our health, and yet many of us avoid it, leading to a sedentary lifestyle. I get that exercise can be intimidating at face value, but it's lifesaving—really.

When it comes to developing healthy exercise habits, getting started is always the hardest part. I don't know about you, but gym anxiety is a real thing for me. For the longest time, I was so scared of going to the gym alone and heading for the weights. I had this idea in my head that people were going to look at me and think I was weird or not executing a movement correctly! Realistically, no one was paying any attention to me in the gym, and these fears were all in my head. Fear truly is a mind-killer. The gym is a place for everyone to better themselves and very much a judgment-free zone.

Whether you prefer to work out in the gym, at home, outside, on your own, or with friends, it doesn't matter—however you decide to exercise, make it a habit. There are a million different ways to exercise and be healthy, and this chapter isn't meant to limit you or tell you what's best. This chapter is for those of you who are overwhelmed and need a starting point to get the minimal but optimal movement for a better life.

No one tells the pro-aging woman what she should be doing to optimize her health, and social media has a whole host of conflicting ideas surrounding what's best for women, longevity, nutrition, exercise, and gut and hormone health. It can be hard to know what's sound advice and what's a trendy hoax.

Let me make this simple for you. Are there exercises or activities that you already do on a regular basis that you enjoy? This can be anything from running, to Pilates, to painting, to baking, to gardening, to camping. "Yes, Dr. Shah. I have hobbies that I enjoy." Okay, great—keep doing those things. Simple. If it fulfills you, brings you joy, and grows your brain, you should do that, especially if it's exercise.

Now, if you have a lot of hobbies that aren't exactly exercise-related, that's okay, too. Here's what you need to know in another easy-to-remember sequence of numbers: 4,3,2,1. I'll break down what this means step-by-step in a moment. When thinking about exercise, it's important to focus on the minimum effort to optimize our health, not the minimum to live. Most of us don't look beyond what we need to live, and it's time to change that. The 4,3,2,1 framework will help you get there and move beyond the bare minimum to better your mind and body as you age. Start small and work your way up to a point where you can incorporate the full 4,3,2,1 in a normal week.

4 TIMES A WEEK: MOVEMENT FOR ENDURANCE

The first element of the 4,3,2,1 framework is engaging in some sort of movement for endurance lasting 45 minutes to an hour at least 4 times a week. For me, this looks like walking, hiking, or jogging. For you, this could look like cycling, swimming, dancing, rowing, playing tennis, or whatever activity gets you moving for an extended period of time.

I chose to call this category "movement for endurance" rather than "cardio" because that word tends to be restrictive and scare people off. The point of engaging in movement for endurance exercises 4 times a week is to promote better mental health, quality of sleep, and decrease your risk of developing cardiovascular disease. It isn't intended to be torture. If you hate running, fantastic. I won't make you include running in your workout routine. The 4,3,2,1 framework is about identifying types of exercise you enjoy and are willing to implement into your regular routine.

Personally, my favorite part of every day is when I get to take a walk outside. I'm known to take meetings with my team over the phone while walking around my neighborhood or on local trails nearby. I try to get between 10,000 and 12,000 steps per day. The great thing about living in Phoenix is that we have access to scenic and challenging trails almost year-round. One of my favorite things in the world is going on a sunrise or sunset hike with my friends or family on one of our local mountain trails—I'll have you know that very few things are more beautiful than an Arizona sunset. Walks in nature as part of my daily routine help quiet my mind and re-center me for the rest of the day. Going for a 45-minute walk in the sunshine is some of the best medicine I can think of, and you won't need a doctor's prescription. Scratch that—consider this my official prescription for you to take a walk outside today.

Quick Pause: The Wonders of Walking

Exercise doesn't always have to be complicated. Walking is often underestimated and not seen as effective as more intense types of movements like running or swimming. Allow me to clear up any misconceptions surrounding the efficacy of walking as a form of exercise. Research on the benefits of walking confirms that this simple movement will improve your health and is a perfectly legitimate form of exercise. Walking for even 30 minutes a day is known to stave off food cravings, ease joint pain, boost immune function, and can even lower the risk of breast cancer.[3]

A recent study from *GeroScience* on the aging process in blue zones and the health benefits of walking found that going for a

30-minute walk 5 days a week will significantly improve health outcomes for those over the age of 50.[4] For many people living in these so-called blue zones, or concentrated areas with higher-than-average life expectancy, walking and other low-impact physical activity is an integral part of daily life that most certainly contributes to improved health and longer lifespans across the board. The researchers conclude that walking is a powerful tool for anti-aging that reduces one's risk of age-related diseases like cardiovascular disease (CVD), hypertension, type 2 diabetes, and certain cancers while also improving pain management, quality of sleep, and mental health. The simple act of walking or engaging in some form of exercise that increases the heart rate half an hour every day will change (and lengthen) your life. You can even consider walking with some form of weight, such as a weighted vest or ankle weights, for added benefits.

The 4,3,2,1 framework is a tool to help you get started, but don't feel discouraged if you can't get 4 days of movement for endurance right away. Four days is the end goal, not the starting point. Begin with incorporating one 45-minute session of movement per week and assess your progress before increasing the frequency. If walking or running is your thing, I recommend trying to get that in within 1 hour of waking up for added benefits. A short 5-to-10-minute walk after meals is great for digestion and lowering blood sugar. My goal for you is 12,500 steps per day throughout perimenopause and menopause for maximum health benefits, including protecting bone health and lowering cortisol. Remember, the best type of walking or running for your health is done outdoors, especially if it's sunny—vitamin D for the win!

3 TIMES A WEEK: BUILDING MUSCLE

Most of the muscle loss women experience as they move through the hormonal continuum happens between the ages of 40 and 50. However, if you're someone who isn't yet there, now is the perfect time to start preservation to stay ahead. The hormone testosterone helps with maintenance and growth of muscles; unfortunately, after the age of 30, testosterone levels begin to drop. A 2019 study found that women in perimenopause and menopause gain body fat percentage and lose lean muscle mass in greater amounts and at a higher rate than at any other period of their life.[5] Even women who have been in good shape their entire lives will notice these changes as they progress along the hormonal continuum—no one is immune to the passage of time and the body's clock along with it. Incorporating weights and stretching into your lifestyle is more important than ever to prevent the negative effects of losing muscle mass and bone density.

That's why it's important to engage in weight-bearing exercises 3 times a week. For those of you who are new to strength training, keep it simple and start with body-weight squats and easy stretching for flexibility. Squats work a wide range of muscles, including some of the largest in your body. One thing to keep in mind: The larger the muscle you're working, the greater the testosterone hit. On the other side of the strength spectrum, flexibility, specifically, is essential for the completion of daily tasks like grabbing clothes out of the dryer or moving a chair in your living room. When working on building strength, flexibility must also be taken into consideration for functional results.

Quick Pause: Suitcase Squats

Allow me to introduce you to one of my favorite exercise movements: the suitcase squat. Simply put, it's the process of performing a squat while holding some kind of weight at your side. This exercise serves to build leg strength, core strength, grip strength, and improve your balance.

For a suitcase squat, you can use dumbbells, kettle bells, cans of soup, or any heavy household item, such as a suitcase as the name implies. Whatever equipment you have at your disposal will work just fine.

Once you have your weights, hold them at your sides.

Keep your feet about shoulder-width apart, whatever feels comfortable. Then, squat down until your thighs are parallel to the ground, forming a right angle at the knee. Drive up with your legs to a standing position. Repeat.

While doing this movement, focus on keeping your arms steady at your sides and your back straight. Try not to curve your shoulders inward under the weight, as this will strain your neck. Keep your core muscles engaged throughout.

Go ahead and give suitcase squats a try. In conjunction with other weight-bearing exercises, you'll start to build muscle and improve your mobility and balance, all things we need to keep moving as we get older.

Maintaining good muscle mass supports mobility, healthy aging, metabolism, and lowered risk of disease or injury. Training your legs, for example, has been shown to specifically improve neurological health. Using the legs for weighted exercise sends signals that are essential for proper brain and nervous system function. A study of women suffering from insomnia, chronic fatigue, depression, and anxiety found that training exercises with body weight contributed significantly to symptom relief.[6]

Researchers from Stanford recommend lifting weights in 4 to 6 reps for 3 to 5 sets for maximized benefit to build and maintain muscle mass during perimenopause.[7] They use the language "near to failure," which means you should be training with weights heavy enough or resistance strong enough that it feels challenging to complete up to 5 sets. This feeling of trying hard, pushing ourselves to the limit, and the muscle aches we feel afterward are signs that our muscles are growing, which is what we want. However, this is not to say that you should be training at maximum effort every time. Exercise caution and do only what feels safe for your body and its ability. If a weight feels too heavy on the first rep, it's okay to switch it out and drop to a lighter weight.

Here's an interesting fact: Muscle memory is a real thing, and it applies to strength training and muscle mass. A randomized controlled trial from the *Scandinavian Journal of Medicine & Science in Sports* found that taking breaks from exercise won't exactly kill your gains in the long-term.[8] The study observed muscle size and strength among a group of people training for 20 consecutive weeks, and a group of people who trained for 10 weeks, took a 10-week break, then came back to training for 10 weeks. This study revealed that within just 5 weeks of returning to training, the group that took a 10-week break was able to fully regain their muscle mass and strength from before the break period. What this means is that if you're doing weight or resistance training regularly and then take a break, you won't lose all the progress you made; however, consistent exercise is always the goal for maximum benefits.

Quick Pause: Adaptive Weight Training

Anyone of any ability can engage in and benefit from weight training. Don't let some of the more intense fitness content on social media scare you into thinking training with weights and building muscle is out of your scope, because it isn't. There are so many ways to adapt weight-bearing exercises to suit all levels of mobility, ability, and health conditions.

A good alternative for weight training that I like to recommend is a weighted vest—you're still moving weights but without putting extra pressure on your joints. For people with osteoporosis, walking or performing aerobic exercises while wearing a vest that is 5 to 10 percent of your total body weight is a wonderful way to get moving without putting yourself at risk of serious injury. Physical therapists and personal trainers are awesome resources for learning to adapt different exercises tailored to your needs.

For me, 3 days per week to build muscle include 2 days spent in the gym doing exercises with free weights, my body weight, and resistance training. I spend the third day in a class setting for either power yoga or Pilates to both promote healthy muscle mass and maintain a sustainable level of flexibility. Yoga and Pilates are low-intensity exercises. This allows you to move your body without a flux in stress hormones; these types of activities can be very helpful in controlling the body's response to stress.

If you're someone who has a lot of anxiety about the gym, I encourage you to join a class of some kind, whether yoga, Pilates, barre, or any other activity that appeals to you and makes you stronger. Fitness classes are a great way to meet people and improve strength and mobility. A personal trainer can also be a significant help for those who are new to using gym equipment or if you have preexisting injuries. If you prefer to fly solo in the gym or work out at home, that's perfectly fine as well. Exercise is not one size fits all, and it takes some trial and error to find what works best for you mentally and physically.

Quick Pause: Yoga Routine for Beginners

If you're new to yoga and want to give it a try, here's a basic flow of poses you can expect at any introductory-level yoga class. These poses are what's known as "restorative yoga" and they are great for stretching and relaxation. The poses as I've listed them will take you less than 20 minutes, but feel free to take as much or little time as you need with each.

1. Easy Seated Breathing: 3 Minutes
- Sit cross-legged with your spine straight.
- Rest your hands on your knees, palms up or down, whatever feels natural.
- Close your eyes and take **slow,** deep breaths in through your nose and out through your mouth.

2. Cat-Cow Stretch: 2 Minutes
- Start in a tabletop position (hands palm down on the mat directly under shoulders, knees under hips).

- Inhale, arch your back, drop your belly, and lift your head (Cow Pose).
- Exhale, round your spine, tuck your chin, and draw your belly in (Cat Pose).
- Repeat slowly, syncing breath with movement. Hold each for as long as feels comfortable.

3. Downward Dog: 2 Minutes
- From the tabletop position, tuck your toes under and lift your hips up and back.
- Keep a slight bend in your knees if needed, and press your hands firmly into the mat.
- Hold and take deep breaths.

4. Standing Forward Fold: 2 Minutes
- Walk your feet forward and fold over your legs, letting your head relax.
- Slightly bend your knees if needed.
- Hold on to opposite elbows, and gently sway side to side if that feels natural.

5. Low Lunge: 2 Minutes (1 minute per side)
- Step one foot forward into a lunge, keeping your back knee down.
- Lift your arms up for a gentle stretch.
- Switch sides and repeat.

6. Seated Forward Fold: 2 Minutes
- Sit with legs extended forward.
- Inhale, reach arms up, then exhale and fold forward, reaching for your toes or shins.
- Keep your back elongated and breathe deeply.

7. Supine Twist: 2 Minutes (1 minute per side)
- Lie on your back and hug your knees into your chest for a tight squeeze, then slowly release the pressure.
- Drop both knees to one side and extend your opposite arm out.
- Hold, then switch sides.

> 8. *Relaxation (Savasana): 3 Minutes*
> - Lie flat on your back, legs slightly apart, arms relaxed at your sides. Palms can be up or down depending on your preference.
> - Close your eyes and focus on your breath, letting your body completely relax. At this point your body should feel looser than it did at the beginning of the session. It's okay if you fall asleep at this stage!

No matter how you choose to exercise, my goal for you is to increase lean muscle, prevent bone loss, and improve balance, flexibility, and mobility for a longer, healthier life. Start by training with weights or resistance once a week, then assess and increase as you're able. When you can get 3 sessions of this type of exercise per week, you're setting yourself up for success and independence later in life.

2 TIMES A WEEK: HEAT THERAPY

Heat therapy has the power to increase your human growth hormone (HGH) by up to 500 percent, which is astounding.[9] What is heat therapy? Great question. Traditionally, this means sauna, but heat therapy also includes participating in hot yoga, sitting in a hot tub or hot bath, exercising in hot weather, or really anything that raises your core body temperature for 15 to 20 minutes at a time.

The growth hormone, somatotropin, is released by the anterior lobe of the pituitary gland and has the power to repair muscles; it's basically behind what we call "beauty sleep." The growth hormone is something that naturally decreases with age, and it isn't something that can be fully replaced by adding more synthetically. There are very few conditions that would cause a doctor to prescribe HGH for patients; these include short bowel syndrome, a growth hormone deficiency, or for muscle loss attributed to HIV.

Let me be very clear that all women will experience a decrease in HGH as they move through the hormonal continuum, which can and often does result in increased abdominal fat, decreased aerobic capacity and muscle mass, and changes in mood or mental health. However, there are even more negative side effects that go along with taking synthetic HGH such as edema, heightened risk of certain cancers, joint pain, and insulin resistance—not to mention that synthetic HGH use without a prescription is banned. You capitalize on your natural growth hormone by simply getting enough sleep and exercise, eating a healthy diet, and by using heat therapy.

The goal is to get 2 days of some form of heat therapy per week to promote the release of HGH along with a whole host of other health benefits as you age. Much of our data surrounding sauna baths and heat therapy comes from Finland, where the use of saunas is commonplace, woven into the fabric of the Finnish lifestyle and culture. In the US and other parts of the world, saunas are not so mainstream (yet), which is why I emphasize that any kind of heat therapy is beneficial—you don't need to go out and buy a sauna for your home or sign up for an expensive gym membership just to access one.

When your core body temperature is elevated through exposure to high temperatures, heat shock proteins are released. These heat shock proteins are stress-induced proteins. So, when your body is feeling heat, it produces these proteins that repair the muscles in our bodies. Regular release of heat shock proteins can be really useful in our long-term health by promoting heart health and preventing cardiovascular disease. The most reliable data we have for supporting the benefits of heat therapy come from Finland, of course, using dry saunas at 167 degrees Fahrenheit 4 or more times a week.

The Mayo Clinic published a review of evidence in 2023, which compiled and analyzed findings from dozens of studies on the impacts of Finnish sauna bathing and other forms of passive heat therapies over time.[10] They concluded that regular sauna use promotes cardiovascular health, decreases adverse effects from inflammation, reduces high systolic blood pressure, and increases one's life span. They noted that frequent sauna bathing helps offset the negative interpersonal factors associated with low socioeconomic status and helps decrease cortisol levels spiked by stress.

More specifically, 8 weeks of consistent sauna use, when paired with exercise, resulted in a mean reduction of around 8mm Hg in systolic blood pressure. The positive effects associated with sauna use are independent of physical activity, yet they can be enhanced when coupled with regular exercise. There's an abundance of evidence to support the notion that for people with impairments who are not able to exercise and for those with limited mobility, regular sauna bathing alone is a useful health intervention for mitigating the risks of various diseases and decreasing mortality.[11] Who doesn't love sitting in the sauna or hot tub every now and then? Not only is it relaxing, but it's also a great health hack.

Quick Pause: Ice Baths and Red-Light Therapy

Some of you may be wondering, "Dr. Shah, what about ice baths?" or "What about red-light therapy?" Those are great questions. The reason why I'm wholeheartedly recommending heat therapy and not cold therapy or red-light therapy is due to the sheer amount of data we have that highlights the benefits of saunas and the relative lack of substantial data that supports long-term benefits of alternative therapies pertaining to cold or photobiomodulation (PBM).

While ice baths reduce inflammation in the short-term and give us an adrenaline rush, cold therapy is a relatively new trend that doesn't yet have the medical data to back it up as a viable option for increasing longevity. Similarly, PBM may be a suitable treatment for certain diseases in the future due to its anti-inflammatory properties (that are yet to be fully understood), but the full implications are still largely unknown.[12] Social media has popularized ice bath and red-light therapy for anti-aging and reducing inflammation, but you should know those are just claims and are lacking in sufficient evidence to be backed by the medical community. The consensus is that these wellness alternatives won't cause you harm, but they also may not bring about the effects you seek. It is highly likely the benefits many people online seem to experience from these therapies is a result of placebo. Sorry, not sorry.

The data we have from Finland and elsewhere on the benefits of sauna is robust, drawn from hundreds of thousands of people contributing to data and studies that are reproducible in other populations. So, there you have it. I'm not scorning ice baths, but I'd much rather have you focus on the benefits I *know* you can achieve through engaging in heat therapy twice a week.

1 TIME A WEEK: SPRINT

The final element of the 4,3,2,1 framework is to sprint once a week. If this made you wrinkle your nose, you're not alone—and hear me out. Most people don't sprint after childhood. Why would you? You may have heard that only 5 percent of adults will ever sprint after the age of 30. When was the last time you gave it absolutely everything you had and full-out sprinted?

As we age, the heart naturally becomes smaller and stiffer with time. This is why heart failure and cardiac disease are more common among older populations. What if I told you that you can reverse or slow the age of your heart? A study took people who were sedentary and put them on a 2-year-long exercise plan.[13] Researchers examined imaging of the participants' hearts and found them to be more flexible and functioning as if their hearts were 20 years younger. The study participants spent a year working up to sprints 1 day a week and using the Norwegian 4x4 training method.

Quick Pause: Norwegian 4x4 Protocol

The Norwegian 4x4 training method is an evidence-based high-intensity interval training (HIIT) regimen designed to increase cardiovascular endurance and improve one's maximum oxygen consumption, or "VO_2 max." When practiced over time, this training method is shown to reverse and slow the age of the heart in both sedentary and active adults.

So, what does it look like? That depends. The Norwegian 4x4 can be adapted to a variety of exercises, really any movements you enjoy that allow you to give maximum effort for a period of 4 minutes. You can utilize this training framework whether you're running, swimming, rowing, cycling, walking uphill, skiing, dancing, or any other high-intensity activity.

Start by warming up for 10 minutes by walking or jogging. Stretching during the warm-up is a good idea as well to prevent injury.

Once you're warmed up, begin your first interval. "Sprint," meaning exert yourself to near maximum effort, for 4 minutes. The goal is to perform at 85 to 95 percent of your maximum heart rate. It is a good idea to wear a heart rate monitor to make sure you are not pushing yourself too hard and to make sure you're at least hitting the target of 85 percent of your maximum heart rate. A simple trick to roughly estimate your maximum heart rate is to subtract your age from 220.

Once you complete your first 4-minute sprint interval, take 3 minutes to rest by walking or continuing to move in some way. Your heart rate should drop to 60 to 70 percent of your maximum heart rate during these 3 minutes. You will want to avoid sitting down between intervals unless you absolutely have to, as it will make you even more tired and causes the heart to exert itself more than if you were to walk.

Repeat this process until you have completed 4 sets of 4-minute sprints (hence the 4x4 name). Afterward, cool down for 5 minutes at the end by walking, jogging, or continuing to move at a mild to moderate intensity.

If you can't complete the full workout on your first try, don't be discouraged. It's incredibly difficult, especially if you aren't used to giving maximum effort during a workout. A helpful tip is to keep a workout journal with a plan, the exercises you completed, and your heart rate during the session. As you improve your physical fitness, you may notice your maximum heart rate will decrease over time as your cardiovascular endurance increases.

What we know from this study and the impact of regular exercise on sedentary bodies is that you can reverse the age of your heart by doing just 1 sprint exercise a week. If you are already exercising regularly and staying active, your heart likely won't be anti-aged by 20 years, but incorporating sprints will help regardless, by slowing the age of the heart and preventing heart attacks or disease. The Norwegian 4x4 training method is just one of many HIIT routines that will work to improve heart health in the long-term.

I'll be honest and say that sprinting is not my favorite thing in the world. However, I understand the long-term benefits of sprinting once a week and have made it a part of my exercise routine. What this typically looks like for me is sprinting for 30 seconds on the treadmill 8 times with 1.5 incline. If you're someone who can't stand treadmills, try sprinting outside on grass or pavement, and time yourself if possible. The aim is to be able to sprint for 30-second bursts totaling up to 4 minutes of maximum effort.

When you start with sprints, it's important to start slow with just 1 and build up from there. Same with heat therapy, especially if you have a medical condition. If you don't already have one, a heart rate monitor is a great tool for gauging your maximum heart rate and making sure you don't overdo it.

What's in it for you?

We all know that a sedentary lifestyle is not ideal for our health. So many of us are sitting for 8 or more hours a day, but research tells us that with each hour of being off your feet, there's a 5 percent increase in premature death risk. That's why getting up and moving at every opportunity is so important. Take a walk at lunch, make phone calls an opportunity for more movement, and don't sit unless you have to.

By moving more, you can expect your risk of disease, back pain symptoms, effects of aging, and more to improve. You don't need to do CrossFit workouts every morning and 3-mile runs after work. Aim for at least 25 to 30 minutes of moderate daily exercise, and yes, walking counts! Your goal after 6 months is to get up to the full 4,3,2,1 every week.

PART III

Putting Everything Together

CHAPTER 9

Moving Through the Continuum: Postmenopause

W HILE I'M WRITING THIS GUIDE for women in perimenopause and menopause, know that these hormonal shifts are a continuum within a greater continuum, and the information I provide here is to make hormonal transitions anywhere on the continuum easier for you. If you're someone who hasn't had a cycle in 10 years, this book is for you, too. And if you're still on your way to perimenopause, here's what you need to know about life after menopause—and what you can look forward to!

Postmenopause is the latter end of the hormonal continuum, a stage that lasts from a year after your period to the end of your life. During this stage, you may continue to experience the same symptoms you experienced in perimenopause or menopause or even develop new symptoms while others dissipate. The best thing you can do to help your body amid postmenopausal hormonal decline is lock in a diet and exercise routine that promotes a healthy gut, strong bones, mobility, and longevity.

I have a postmenopausal patient in her sixties, let's call her Julie. She first came to me because she had been hearing so much about menopause, but she was really confused about what to do with her nutrition after menopause. "Is what I should be doing during postmenopause the same as in menopause? No one really talks about what happens once you've gone through it already." Julie didn't feel equipped with sufficient knowledge during her menopausal journey, and she felt lost, unsure about where to turn now that menopause was behind her. I spoke with her about different options for changing her diet to improve her gut health, and I counseled her on trying to identify her gifts by spending time with the right people, spending more time outdoors and staying active, and eating the right foods.

We changed her morning routine to include a short walk in the sun (weather permitting) and 20 minutes for journaling to add a buffer to her demanding day ahead. I recommended she eat more protein and fiber in her first meal, which she often doesn't eat until closer to noon. She used to skip meals all the way to dinner, so our goal was to add a meal earlier in the day, a snack at 3 p.m., and then dinner between 5 and 6 p.m. I also gave her a goal of going to sleep around the same time each night and waking up around the same time each day.

After 3 months of working together, Julie told me that she has never felt better, that she's picked up new hobbies she's super passionate about, and she spends a lot of her free time with good friends, getting outside more, and making walks part of her routine. She even started using the sauna a few times each week. During one of our appointments, she told me that the cloud of uncertainty and helplessness she experienced during menopause was gone, and that she's now able to live out her potential, something she couldn't see before.

This is why I do what I do and why I will never stop advocating for more awareness regarding women's health across every stage of the hormonal continuum. It's never too late to change your life through more intentional, healthy choices.

Quick Pause: The Grandmother Effect

Here's a fun fact: The majority of animals do not live past menopause; only a few species, humans obviously one of them, experience life after their reproductive years. The grandmother effect (also known as the grandmother hypothesis) describes the theory that women were naturally selected to live past menopause due to the vital roles we hold in our communities outside of procreation.[1] Think about it: Women literally survive organ failure. Menopause, the permanent cessation of menses, is the process of our ovaries ceasing to function–gradual reproductive organ failure.

Generally, organ failure in any being is fatal, and yet women live decades after our reproductive organs are senescent. How amazing is that? This idea has posed something of an evolutionary conundrum to researchers as it contradicts many theories surrounding how and why animals evolve. If the biological purpose of women is to reproduce, why is our reproductive window short relative to our lifespan? The academic consensus surrounding this question supports the notion that women evolved because they were needed, especially after they were done having children.[2] As humans began to transition from hunting and gathering to cultivating crops, communities needed all hands on deck to maintain the food supply. Infants cannot harvest vegetables or prepare dinner, but grandmothers can. Throughout human history, grandmothers, matronly figures, and elder women in communities were vital for their roles as providers, vessels of knowledge from generations past, and stewards for future generations to come.

This idea rings true today. Women are vital to the advancement of society beyond serving a biological function. Life does not end at menopause for a reason–you can accomplish whatever you put your mind to at any age. Whether you realize it yet or not, your age or ability to have children does not define you or the value you bring to the world.

Considering that the average woman spends about a third of her life postmenopause, it's crucial that we understand the importance of the gut-brain-hormone connection even after we've progressed through menopause into postmenopause glory. You can grow your brain, build muscle, learn new things, start a new career, or enter a new relationship at any age, after all. It's never too late for big life changes, and it's never too late to learn how to take control of your health.

Around 60 percent of postmenopausal women are still having symptoms that reflect perimenopause—headaches, nausea, you know the drill.[3] Why is this the case? Being "postmenopausal" means you haven't had a period in over a year, but your reproductive hormones don't suddenly disappear into thin air along with your cycle. It takes time for your hormones to transition and stabilize once your cycle stops, which means you may continue to experience many of the same symptoms as you did in earlier stages of the continuum. These symptoms should lessen over time and eventually stop.

Congratulations! There's no need to spend hundreds of more dollars on tampons, pads, and other period products! While being postmenopausal means you gradually have less of those pesky menopause symptoms, this doesn't mean you can ditch the awesome lifestyle habits you've so diligently practiced these past years. Now more than ever, these healthy habits will come in handy to lengthen your life and prevent disease.

The low estrogen levels that come after menopause put postmenopausal women at greater risk of osteoporosis and cardiovascular disease.[4] Your reproductive hormones play a key role in keeping your heart and bones healthy, and when those hormones dramatically decrease, you need to be able to compensate through nutrition and exercise to lower your risk of losing bone density or developing cardiovascular disease.

HEALTHY LIVING IN POSTMENOPAUSE

A compelling point I noticed through my research and speaking to women is that we need more points of connection in our lives to thrive, especially at older ages. Humans are inherently social beings, and the impact our social lives have on our physical health is profound. There's such power that comes from spending time with others in person, especially today when many of us spend a substantial chunk of time in front of screens.

Knowing this, I created a wellness retreat designed for women of all ages to come together, to learn about their bodies and nutrition, and to connect. Forty women joined us at the retreat, and at first I didn't know their ages, why they signed up, or what they wanted out of the experience. I sent an email with a few questions to get to know these women a little more prior to meeting them in person, and the responses were fascinating.

The women in the group ranged from mid-twenties to older than 70, and their reasons for attending were all different. One woman wanted to understand the link between her diet and hormones, while another wanted a space to socialize with other women and share about their experiences. Someone was struggling with debilitating menopause symptoms, and another had already gone through menopause and wanted to work on self-care strategies to calm her mind and body.

By the end of the retreat, we went over everything in the Shah Protocol from my nutrition framework, the science behind hormones, self-care, exercise, mental health, and so much more. It was a gift beyond measure to meet these women and to observe friendships blossom from connecting with others about prioritizing our health. I'm certain that each woman left the retreat feeling more in tune with her body and empowered to be in the driver's seat of her health and nutrition. On a personal note, I left the retreat feeling reinvigorated and even more inspired to keep sharing what I know so that women everywhere could feel like their most powerful selves. I felt especially inspired by the postmenopausal women at the retreat—they were vibrant, active, and strong women who exemplified everything I want for myself postmenopause, and they were a reminder that life doesn't stop when your ability to menstruate does.

Conversations surrounding women's health, perimenopause, menopause, and postmenopause are not just for women in their thirties or forties. This is a conversation for everyone. If you've walked through a bookstore recently or searched online for books about gut health, you may notice that most books on this subject are by men, and there is little mention of the link between gut health and the hormonal continuum. That's where I come into the picture.

I have dedicated my life to understanding the intersection of the gut microbiome, nutrition, and women's health and how these affect our hormones. For far too long, most women have moved across the hormonal continuum in the dark and not knowing what was happening to their bodies. Menopause isn't like going through puberty; there's no health teacher equipped with an embarrassing video and pamphlet to explain the wonders of the aging female body; there's no group Q&A session with fellow women who are equally confused and scared about the new changes they're experiencing (well, unless you attend a retreat like mine!).

As a society, we don't talk about women's health enough, and we definitely don't discuss what happens when our cycles change, then stop. I'm doing everything I can to change that narrative, to cut through the silence and the confusion, and to make conversations and awareness surrounding women's health and aging mainstream.

While your postmenopausal body may have different needs than those of your younger self, the essential pillars of a healthy lifestyle remain the same:

- A diet of whole foods and vital nutrients guided by the 30–30–3
- Regular exercise
- A strong gut-brain connection
- Good sleep hygiene
- Time spent in nature
- Hobbies and activities that enrich your life
- A strong support network
- Stress management strategies

I've spoken about each of these elements at length (refer to part II), and they apply just as much in life postmenopause as they did in perimenopause. While these core aspects of healthy living remain the same, there may be some changes you need to make to address ongoing symptoms, new symptoms that may pop up, and the mental and physical tolls of aging. For example, your doctor may recommend a form of MHT or introduce a supplement to your diet to combat the loss of bone density. Maybe you're suddenly having trouble sleeping. This could be a sign that you need to adapt your old routine to meet the needs of the new you. It may be hard to pick up on these changes at first, but the sooner you're able to identify your postmenopausal body's needs and revise your lifestyle habits, the better your experience will be. Aging doesn't have to be scary!

CHECKING IN WITH THE NEW YOU

In my role as a medical professional and content creator, I've become very skilled at taking health concepts that are highly complex and challenging to communicate in plain English and creating coherent, easy-to-remember mnemonics, acronyms, and tools for understanding your health. Before the wellness retreat, I wanted a way to distill everything you needed to know about the gut-brain-hormone connection into a short exercise. I came up with a wellness checklist in the form of a body scan and found it to be a highly effective way to get women thinking about the interconnectedness of gut health, hormones, nutrition, mental health, and physical activity. This checklist can be something you write down in your diary or it can serve as a mental check-in for you throughout the week. By now, I'm sure you've already been thinking a lot about the elements we're about to discuss, but I want you to think of this as a postmenopause check-in. For those still a long way to postmenopause, you can complete the scan now and use it as a baseline for later, when your hormones reach their low point—dog-ear this section for a later date and complete the scan again, then compare.

Start with the brain. How are we doing today? When was the last time you did a mental check-in with yourself? Sit (or stand, or walk, doesn't make a difference to me) for a moment and reflect; allow yourself to *feel* how you're feeling. Deep breath. Now, ask yourself if the way you're feeling is influenced by some of the choices you've made recently, better or worse. How's your sleep? What's your relationship with your phone like? Did you get a chance to go for a walk today? Did you take your magnesium and omega-3? Having regular check-ins with yourself about your health and how you're feeling can go a long way in helping you identify when something is or isn't working for you and when you need to consider making some sort of lifestyle change, big or small.

Let's move on to the heart. Do you have a pulse? Okay, awesome! Moving on—kidding. But seriously, this part of the body scan is focused on your cardiovascular health and movement. Think about your average day and how many steps you take. Some of you may already know this data from a smartwatch or fitness tracker, while others may need to take a moment to estimate. The average American walks between 3,000 and 4,000 steps a day, which is less than 2 miles—we can and should be moving more. Further, doing 1 "sprint" per week can slow the age of the heart. Maybe the word "cardio" puts a bad taste in your mouth. I get it. Really, any aerobic exercise you can muster at least once a week will help promote heart health.

This next part of the scan is harder to visualize, but picture your hormones. As you know, estrogen levels begin to decrease during perimenopause. This is natural. However, there are things we can do to combat natural hormone decline. You know that vitamin D levels drop during perimenopause, so start taking a vitamin D supplement if you haven't already. As a bonus, regular sauna use can help with hormonal imbalances, particularly through lowering cortisol levels. If you're currently on MHT, do you feel that your symptoms have lessened, or are you experiencing new ones?

Moving on to the gut, my favorite part of the body scan! I've said it before and I'll say it again, the gut microbiome is integral to every aspect of your health. The first step in improving your gut health is through, you guessed it, food! Refer to the chapter on the 30–30–3 framework for detailed information on how you should be eating to fuel your body, fix your gut, and live longer. When your gut health improves, so, too, will your hormone health, mental health, and more, especially as you age.

The last part of the scan is to visualize your bones, the skeleton holding your body together. When we talk about bone health, most of you might jump to the conclusion that taking a calcium supplement will help prevent bone loss. While that isn't exactly wrong, it's more complex than that. Think back to our discussion of vitamin D and how women in menopause, across the board, present with low levels of it. Remember also that women postmenopause have a greater risk of osteoporosis and arthritis. There is a direct link here. Taking a vitamin D supplement can help prevent loss of bone density and so can weight training. This isn't to say every woman should hit the gym and start deadlifting 300 pounds right off the bat, but we know that incorporating weight-resistance training at least once a week can help build and maintain lean muscle to promote stronger bones, potentially avoiding the risk of osteoporosis altogether.

I encourage you to use this body scan every so often to do a self-assessment of your health and to stay in touch with your body and notice the changes you may not have picked up on otherwise. We can improve our health only when we know what to focus on and what we're doing right. As always, consult your doctor on any major lifestyle changes, and know that postmenopause does not have to be the worst years of your life. Crazy, right? You can improve your hormone health and make your aging journey a smoother one.

THE BIG PICTURE

No matter where you are on your journey along the hormonal continuum, there are small changes you can start making today that will improve your gut health, the mind-gut-hormone connection, and increase your lifespan. It isn't just about being "healthier" this week or this month—it's about understanding your body, listening to its needs, and having the ability to make conscious decisions and develop positive lifestyle habits that will boost your quality of life in the long term.

The cancer we develop at 50 actually starts at 30. Heart disease at 60 started in our twenties. Our fragile bones at 80 started losing density at 40. Keep in mind that the person you want to be in the future begins with the work you do and the choices you make for yourself today.

What you eat, the sunlight you get, how active you are, the people you surround yourself with—these things can age you 20 years or increase your lifespan by 20 years, seriously. When you master your nutrition and optimize your brain-gut health, you can discover gifts that you never knew you had.

I don't believe in the old ways of gaslighting women for what they are feeling, keeping them in the dark about what's happening to their bodies as they age. By lifting all women and giving them the tools they need to optimize their health, we can live to see a better version of our world, one that values women beyond their ability to reproduce.

To anyone out there afraid of getting older, terrified of menopause, or dreading what comes next: You got this. Just because you're another year older and just because your hormones aren't what they were in your twenties doesn't mean you have to stop living for yourself and doing what you love. At a certain age, you realize that the "prize" is not expensive clothing, a fast car, or a fancy house; the real prize is a strong, healthy body, a clear and sharp mind, a solid network of supportive friends and family, and the freedom to do what you want. Age is just a number, and I firmly believe the best is yet to come.

CHAPTER 10

The Shah Protocol in Action

H ERE IS SOMETHING I HAVEN'T shared with many people: When I was growing up as an Indian immigrant living in America, I didn't see any women around me pursuing their dreams. Mind you, I think my mother and many of the women in my family and social circle were really happy, yet they often talked about all the things they wanted to do that they never pursued. They had to devote their energy to other important aspects of their life such as getting married, starting a family, and beginning a new life in a new country.

When it came time to sit down and decide what to do with my life, I started to think about the women who came before me, the women I grew up with and looked up to very much. Should I do the same as they did? Should I put off my career plans for a family? I knew deep down I wanted to help people, and I was drawn to medicine because it would give me the ability to make a difference. But was it my place to take on the lifelong challenge and commitment necessary to be a doctor?

Luckily, my dad recognized the deeper purpose of my life within me early on, and he was so supportive, always urging me to go for it. He assured me that this was a new country with new opportunities and boundless potential to make a mark. I really have him to thank for giving me the confidence I needed to commit to myself and my dreams of helping others. I often look back at my young self at a crossroads, unsure of the right way forward, and I'm infinitely grateful for the way my father pushed me to embrace the bright future this new country offered, his reason for bringing our family here. He believed in me and my right to get an education and my ability to succeed in anything I set my mind to. I believe that all women with the right support system and drive can pursue their dreams and succeed, whether that means getting a college degree, embarking upon a fulfilling career, taking care of loved ones or becoming a great mother, traveling the world, learning new skills and trying new hobbies, or more likely a combination of these things. I firmly believe women can live a full and exciting life and feel good in their bodies along the way.

Part of my lifelong mission to help others in my role as a medical doctor is my specific mission to help women everywhere realize their potential and give them the knowledge they need to take control of their path on the hormonal continuum. Women are magnificent, wonderfully unique—each and every one of us. The way we walk through the world is not the same as our neighbor, and yet one commonality that unites us is the hormonal continuum and our ability to take control of it and our lives for the better.

While medical research on women in perimenopause has a very long way to go, we know so much more about our bodies now than our grandmothers did. It is up to us to take advantage of our understanding of the gut-brain-hormone axis and make conscious decisions toward building a lifestyle optimized for longevity. By now, you've read about the importance of nutrition, the gut microbiome, and strategies you can implement to help manage the long list of perimenopausal symptoms. But how does it all fit together?

The following is a full 7-day guide to living the Shah Protocol complete with recipes aligned with the 30–30–3 (see chapter 3) for a standard diet that includes meat and dairy; for vegan and grain-free options, feel free to swap any of the meal suggestions in the plan with meals from the vegan and grain-free recipe sections to suit your dietary needs. Or, if you eat meat and dairy but are wanting to try some plant-based options, the vegan recipes are perfect places to start. Feel free to follow the protocol exactly or jump around and take what you need when you need it. This book and the following guide are your tools for making the most of your hormonal continuum and living healthier, longer.

7-DAY PROTOCOL

Day 1

Start your day from 6:00–7:00 a.m.

Challenge: Get outside within an hour of waking. Go for a walk, sit on the porch with your coffee, read a book outside, just do something to help you get the day started right. If the weather isn't so great, open a window for fresh air and try to let sunlight in.

Breakfast: Cheesy Scrambled Eggs with Veggies and Toast
Aim to eat breakfast from 9:00–10:00 a.m.

Lunch: Grilled Chicken Salad with Avocado, Quinoa, and Kimchi
Aim to eat lunch between 1:00–3:00 p.m.

Snack (as needed): Greek Yogurt with Mixed Berries and Walnuts

Exercise: 40 minutes of walking; 45 minutes of weight or resistance training

Dinner: Grilled Salmon with Roasted Brussels Sprouts, Sweet Potato Wedges, Lentils, and Steamed Asparagus
Aim to eat dinner between 5:00–7:00 p.m.
Take a short walk outside after dinner, even if it's just 10 minutes.
Dim lights and turn off devices by 9:00 p.m.
Plan to get to sleep between 9:00–10:30 p.m.

Day 2

Start your day between 6:00–7:00 a.m.

Challenge: No screens 30 minutes before bed. The goal is 1 hour without screens before sleep, but getting even 30 minutes will help you fall asleep more quickly. Bonus: Limit your total social media scrolling time to only 30 minutes for the whole day.

Breakfast: Cottage Egg Scramble with Veggies and Hummus Toast
Aim to eat breakfast between 9:00–10:00 a.m.

Lunch: Grilled Chicken Breast with Roasted Sweet Potato and Green Beans, Salad with Kimchi
Aim to eat lunch between 1:00–3:00 p.m.

Snack (as needed): Greek Yogurt with Chia Seeds and Raspberries

Exercise: 30 minutes of walking; 45 minutes of yoga or a low-intensity body-weight workout; 20 minutes of heat therapy

Dinner: Baked Salmon with Steamed Broccoli, Quinoa, and Roasted Brussels Sprouts

Aim to eat dinner between 5:00–7:00 p.m.

Take a short walk outside after dinner, even if it's just 10 minutes.

Dim lights and turn off devices by 9:00 p.m.

Plan to get to sleep between 9:00–10:30 p.m.

Day 3

Start your day between 6:00–7:00 a.m.

Challenge: Do something that makes you happy today. Find something that you love to do—a physical activity, a creative hobby, going out with a friend, or anything else that you love—and take at least an hour to do it simply because it brings you joy. It can be difficult to remember to take time for ourselves throughout the week, so use this time to unwind and focus on you.

Breakfast: Berry Yogurt Parfait with Boiled Eggs

Aim to eat breakfast between 9:00–10:00 a.m.

Lunch: Turkey and Avocado Wrap with Roasted Cauliflower and Kimchi

Aim to eat lunch between 1:00–3:00 p.m.

Snack (as needed): Apple with Almond Butter

Exercise: 40 minutes of walking; four 30-second sprints, 2-minute rests in between; 30 minutes of weight or resistance training

Dinner: Grilled Shrimp and Zoodle Salad with Sauerkraut

Aim to eat dinner between 5:00–7:00 p.m.

Take a short walk outside after dinner, even if it's just 10 minutes.

Dim lights and turn off devices by 9:00 p.m.

Plan to get to sleep between 9:00–10:30 p.m.

Day 4

Start your day between 6:00–7:00 a.m.

Challenge: Try a new exercise! You can try a new machine or piece of equipment at the gym, take a class you've never taken before, complete a new workout routine, or experiment with a variation of an exercise you already do. Exercise doesn't have to be boring or the same every time.

Breakfast: Protein Smoothie and Whole-Grain Toast with Almond Butter and Sauerkraut

Aim to eat breakfast between 9:00–10:00 a.m.

Lunch: Grilled Chicken Salad with Quinoa and Kimchi

Aim to eat lunch between 1:00–3:00 p.m.

Snack (as needed): Greek Yogurt with Mixed Berries and Chia Seeds

Exercise: 30 minutes of walking; 45 minutes of weight or resistance training; 20 minutes of heat therapy

Dinner: Baked Salmon with Roasted Brussels Sprouts, Mashed Sweet Potato, and Steamed Green Beans

Aim to eat dinner between 5:00–7:00 p.m.

Take a short walk outside after dinner, even if it's just 10 minutes.

Dim lights and turn off devices by 9:00 p.m.

Plan to get to sleep between 9:00–10:30 p.m.

Day 5

Start your day between 6:00–7:00 a.m.

Challenge: Have your last caffeinated beverage 10 hours before you plan to go to bed. Tip: Don't eat within 1 hour of going to bed.

Breakfast: Breakfast Burrito with Black Beans, Chicken, and Sauerkraut

Aim to eat breakfast between 9:00–10:00 a.m.

Lunch: Turkey Burger with Sweet Potato, Broccoli, and Kimchi Salad

Aim to eat lunch between 1:00–3:00 p.m.

Snack (as needed): Chia Pudding with Raspberries and Walnuts

Exercise: 45 minutes of walking; 45 minutes of yoga or low-intensity body-weight workout

Dinner: Grilled Cod with Mashed Cauliflower, Roasted Zucchini, and Steamed Asparagus

Aim to eat dinner between 5:00–7:00 p.m.

Take a short walk outside after dinner, even if it's just 10 minutes.

Dim lights and turn off devices by 9:00 p.m.

Plan to get to sleep between 9:00–10:30 p.m.

Day 6

Start your day between 6:00–7:00 a.m.

Challenge: Practice mindful breathing for 10 minutes today. Whether it's before bed, during a break, or while you're on your walk, take some time to sit quietly and focus on your breath. Breathe in for a count of 4, hold for 4, and exhale for 4. This simple practice can help reduce stress and increase clarity throughout your day.

Breakfast: Feta Veggie Omelet with Avocado, Toast, and Yogurt

Aim to eat breakfast between 9:00–10:00 a.m.

Lunch: Turkey Lettuce Wraps with Hummus, Quinoa, and Sauerkraut

Aim to eat lunch between 1:00–3:00 p.m.

Snack (as needed): Cottage Cheese with Chia Seeds and Mixed Berries

Exercise: 40 minutes of walking; 45 minutes of weight or resistance training

Dinner: Baked Cod with Roasted Sweet Potatoes, Kale, and Kimchi

Aim to eat dinner between 5:00–7:00 p.m.

Take a short walk outside after dinner, even if it's just 10 minutes.

Dim lights and turn off devices by 9:00 p.m.

Plan to get to sleep between 9:00–10:30 p.m.

Day 7

Start your day between 6:00–7:00 a.m.

Challenge: Set a small goal for the day and accomplish it. It could be as simple as organizing a drawer, finishing a book chapter, or sending an email you've been putting off. Acting on a small goal can create a sense of achievement and boost your confidence for bigger tasks ahead.

Breakfast: Scrambled Tofu with Spinach, Mushrooms, and Toast
Aim to eat breakfast between 9:00–10:00 a.m.

Lunch: Tuna Salad with Avocado, Chickpeas, and Kimchi
Aim to eat lunch between 1:00–3:00 p.m.

Snack (as needed): Apple with Almond Butter and Pumpkin Seeds

Exercise: 30 minutes of walking; 45 minutes of yoga or a low-intensity body-weight workout; 20 minutes of heat therapy

Dinner: Grilled Chicken with Roasted Cauliflower, Brown Rice, and Sauerkraut
Aim to eat dinner between 5:00–7:00 p.m.

Take a short walk outside after dinner, even if it's just 10 minutes.

Dim lights and turn off devices by 9:00 p.m.

Plan to get to sleep between 9:00–10:30 p.m.

Fermented Vegetables

Probiotic pro tip: Make your own fermented vegetables and never stress about getting your 3 daily servings of probiotics again. It's way easier than you think.

Ingredients:
- **Vegetables:** Choose fresh, firm options like cauliflower, radishes, carrots, and green beans.
- **Brine:** Dissolve 1 to 3 tablespoons of sea salt in 4 cups of nonchlorinated water.
- **Flavorings (optional):** Garlic cloves, chilies, and peppercorns can add extra zest.

Equipment:
- Clean glass jar with a lid
- Nonmetallic utensils
- Fermentation weight or a small ziplock bag filled with brine to keep vegetables submerged

Steps:
1. **Sterilize the jar:** Wash the jar and lid thoroughly with warm, soapy water, then rinse with nonchlorinated water to avoid contaminants.
2. **Prepare the brine:** Mix sea salt into water until fully dissolved.
3. **Prepare the vegetables:** Wash and cut them into desired sizes.
4. **Pack the jar:** Place vegetables and any optional flavorings into the jar, leaving about 1 inch of headspace.
5. **Add the brine:** Pour the brine over the vegetables, ensuring they are completely submerged to prevent mold growth.
6. **Weigh down:** Use a fermentation weight or a brine-filled ziplock bag to keep the vegetables submerged.
7. **Seal and ferment:** Close the jar lid loosely to allow gases to escape, or cover with a cloth secured by a rubber band. Let it ferment at room temperature, away from direct sunlight, for 2 to 3 days.
8. **Check for readiness:** Look for bubbles and a tangy aroma, indicating active fermentation. Taste to ensure the desired flavor and texture.
9. **Refrigerate:** Once fermented to your liking, seal the jar tightly and store it in the refrigerator to slow fermentation.

Tips:
- **Cleanliness:** Ensure all equipment and hands are clean to prevent unwanted bacteria.
- **Temperature:** Maintain a consistent room temperature; cooler environments may require longer fermentation periods.
- **Monitoring:** Check daily for signs of fermentation and to ensure vegetables remain submerged.

Recipes

BREAKFAST

Cheesy Scramble with Spinach, Toast, and Sauerkraut

The perfect start to your day with plenty of protein, fiber, and probiotics to fuel your busy routine.

Yield: 1 serving | Total Time: 15 minutes
Calories: 490 | Protein: 31g | Fiber: 7g

3 large eggs
1 teaspoon extra-virgin olive oil
2 tablespoons shredded cheddar cheese
1 cup fresh packaged spinach
5–6 cherry tomatoes, halved
1 slice whole-grain bread
1 tablespoon almond butter
¼ cup sauerkraut
Sea salt and ground black pepper

1. In a small bowl, whisk the eggs until well beaten. Heat a nonstick sauté pan over medium heat and lightly coat it with the olive oil. Pour in the eggs and cook, stirring gently, until the eggs are scrambled and fully cooked through, about 5 to 10 minutes. Fold in the shredded cheese and allow it to melt. Set the scrambled eggs aside in a clean, small bowl.
2. In the same pan, sauté the spinach about 1 to 2 minutes until it starts to wilt. Add the cherry tomatoes and cook for another 1 to 2 minutes until the tomatoes soften. Remove from the heat.
3. While the eggs and veggies are cooking, toast the whole-grain bread to your liking. Spread the almond butter on top of the warm toast.

4. Serve the scrambled eggs with the sautéed spinach and cherry tomatoes on the side. Add the toast with almond butter next to the eggs. Serve the sauerkraut in a small dish or on the side to complete the meal.

SERVING/STORAGE:
Best served immediately.
Scrambled eggs and sautéed vegetables can be stored in an airtight container in the fridge for up to 2 days and reheated gently.
Toast and almond butter should be made fresh.
After opening, sauerkraut should be stored in the fridge and will last for 1 to 2 months.

Cottage Scramble with Veggies, Hummus Toast, and Sauerkraut

A healthy breakfast packed full of protein, fiber, probiotics, and deliciousness to get you going in the morning.

Yield: 1 serving | Total Time: 15–20 minutes
Calories: 407 | Protein: 32g | Fiber: 7g

3 large eggs
1 teaspoon extra-virgin olive oil (for sautéing)
1 cup chopped kale
½ bell pepper, diced
¼ cup cottage cheese
1 slice whole-grain bread
1 tablespoon hummus
¼ cup sauerkraut
Sea salt and ground black pepper

1. In a small bowl, whisk the eggs until well beaten. In a nonstick skillet, heat the extra-virgin olive oil over medium heat. Add the kale and bell pepper to the skillet and sauté for 2 to 3 minutes until the veggies begin to soften. Pour in the eggs and scramble. Add the cottage cheese to melt and continue until cooked through, about 5 to 10 minutes.

2. While the eggs are cooking, toast the bread to your liking. Spread the hummus on top of the warm toast.
3. Serve the scrambled egg mixture alongside the toast. Add the sauerkraut to complete the meal.

SERVING/STORAGE:

Best served immediately. Hummus toast is best enjoyed fresh.

Scrambled eggs and veggies can be stored for up to 2 days in the fridge.

Sauerkraut can be stored in the fridge for 1 to 2 months.

Yogurt Parfait with Berries and Boiled Eggs

A simple, high-protein breakfast full of fiber that will curb your cravings without making you feel bloated.

Yield: 1 serving | Total Time: 15 minutes
Calories: 375 | Protein: 35g | Fiber: 9g

1 cup unsweetened Greek yogurt
¼ cup granola
1 tablespoon chia seeds
¼ cup mixed berries (e.g., strawberries, blueberries, raspberries)
2 large eggs

1. In a medium bowl or glass, layer the Greek yogurt, granola, chia seeds, and mixed berries. Top the parfait with an extra sprinkle of granola or berries if desired.
2. In a small saucepan, cover the eggs with water. Bring to a boil, then reduce the heat to low and simmer for 9 to 10 minutes. Remove the eggs from the water and let them cool. Peel the eggs and serve on the side.

SERVING/STORAGE:

A parfait is best served fresh but can be layered ahead and stored for 1 day (the berries may soften).

Boiled eggs can be made ahead and stored unpeeled in the fridge for up to 1 week.

Protein Smoothie and Whole-Grain Toast with Almond Butter and Sauerkraut

This is a quick-and-easy breakfast option when you're in a hurry to get your day started.

Yield: 1 serving | Total Time: 10 minutes
Calories: 487 | Protein 34g | Fiber 8g

    1 scoop protein powder (your choice of flavor)
    1 cup almond milk
    ½ banana
    1 cup packaged spinach
    1 tablespoon peanut butter
    1 slice whole-grain bread
    1 tablespoon almond butter
    ¼ cup sauerkraut

1. In a blender, combine the protein powder, almond milk, banana, spinach, and peanut butter. Blend until smooth and creamy. Add more almond milk if needed to reach your desired consistency.
2. While you are blending the smoothie, toast the bread to your liking. Spread the almond butter on the warm toast.
3. Pour your protein smoothie into a glass and enjoy it alongside the toast with sauerkraut.

SERVING/STORAGE:
    Smoothies are best fresh but can be stored for up to 1 day (shake before drinking).
    Toast should be made fresh.
    After opening, sauerkraut keeps for 1 to 2 months refrigerated.

Breakfast Burrito with Black Beans, Chicken, and Sauerkraut

A classic breakfast with a probiotic twist: full of nutrient-dense foods without compromising on flavor!

Yield: 1 serving | Total Time: 30 minutes
Calories: 335 | Protein: 43g | Fiber: 12g

3-ounce chicken breast
¼ cup egg whites
Cooking spray or 1 teaspoon extra-virgin olive oil
Sea salt and ground black pepper
¼ cup black beans
1 small whole-wheat tortilla
¼ cup sauerkraut
1 tablespoon salsa (optional)

1. Grill or cook the chicken using a grill, pan, or bake it in the oven until it reaches an internal temperature of 165°F (about 6 to 7 minutes per side on a grill or stovetop). Once cooked, slice the chicken into bite-size pieces or strips and set aside.
2. In a small bowl, whisk the egg whites. Heat a nonstick skillet over medium heat and lightly coat with cooking spray or oil. Pour the egg mixture into the skillet and cook for about 3 to 4 minutes, stirring gently, until the eggs are scrambled and fully cooked through. Season with a pinch of salt and pepper to taste.
3. If you're using canned black beans, drain and rinse them under cold water to remove excess sodium. In a small saucepan, heat the black beans over medium heat for about 2 to 3 minutes until warmed through. Stir occasionally.
4. In a large skillet over medium heat, heat the tortilla for about 20 to 30 seconds on each side until warm and slightly toasted. You can also microwave it for about 10 to 15 seconds.
5. Lay the warm tortilla flat on a plate. Add the scrambled eggs in the center of the tortilla. Top with the grilled chicken pieces, warm black beans, sauerkraut, and salsa (if using). Fold the sides of the tortilla inward and then roll it up tightly from the bottom to enclose all the fillings.

6. Slice the burrito in half, if desired, and serve immediately. Optionally, you can serve it with extra salsa or avocado on the side for extra flavor.

SERVING/STORAGE:

Burritos are best served fresh but can be stored for up to 1 day in the fridge if wrapped tightly.

Cooked chicken and beans can be stored for up to 4 days in the fridge.

After opening, sauerkraut keeps for 1 to 2 months refrigerated.

Feta Veggie Omelet with Avocado, Toast, and Greek Yogurt

A Greek-inspired omelet with healthy fats and tons of protein. Not only is it a great breakfast option, but it's a tasty meal for any time of day.

Yield: 1 serving | Total Time: 15 minutes
Calories: 495 | Protein: 31g | Fiber: 8g

3 large eggs
1 teaspoon extra-virgin olive oil
¼ cup diced bell peppers
¼ cup diced onions
¼ cup packaged spinach
2 tablespoons feta cheese
Sea salt and ground black pepper
1 slice whole-grain bread
½ cup unsweetened Greek yogurt
½ avocado, sliced

1. In a small bowl, whisk the eggs until well beaten.
2. In a large nonstick skillet, heat the extra-virgin olive oil over medium heat. Add the diced peppers, onions, and spinach, and sauté for 1 to 2 minutes.
3. Pour in the eggs and cook, gently stirring, for 5 to 10 minutes until the eggs are fully cooked. Add the feta cheese, let it melt, and season with salt and pepper. Set aside.
4. Toast the whole-grain bread to your liking.

5. Scoop the Greek yogurt into a small bowl.
6. Serve the omelet with avocado slices on the side.

SERVING/STORAGE:

Best served immediately.

The omelet can be refrigerated for up to 2 days and reheated gently.

The toast and avocado should be prepped fresh.

Greek yogurt stores well in the fridge for 5 to 7 days after opening.

Scrambled Tofu with Spinach, Mushrooms, and Whole-Grain Toast

Plant-based and guaranteed to get your morning started off right. The perfect combination of protein, fiber, and flavor.

Yield: 1 serving | Total Time: 10–12 minutes
Calories: 490 | Protein: 30g | Fiber: 10g

1 tablespoon extra-virgin olive oil
¼ cup sliced button mushrooms
½ cup chopped spinach
1 cup crumbled firm tofu
Sea salt and ground black pepper
¼ cup shredded cheddar cheese (optional)
1 slice whole-grain bread
¼ cup unsweetened Greek yogurt

1. In a large nonstick skillet, heat the extra-virgin olive oil over medium heat and cook the mushrooms and spinach for 2 to 3 minutes. Add the crumbled tofu and cook, stirring occasionally, for 5 minutes. Season with salt and pepper and fold in shredded cheese (if desired).
2. Toast the whole-grain bread to your liking.
3. Scoop the Greek yogurt into a small dish for probiotics.

SERVING/STORAGE:

Best if fresh.

Tofu scramble can be stored for 3 to 4 days and reheated.

Tofu Scramble with Veggies, Sprouted Grain Toast, Sauerkraut, and Edamame

A vegan breakfast scramble infused with turmeric, a superfood in its own right. This breakfast option is an immunity booster packed with great nutrients.

Yield: 1 serving | Total Time: 15–20 minutes
Calories: 438 | Protein: 35g | Fiber: 15g

1 cup firm tofu, crumbled
1 teaspoon ground turmeric
Sea salt and ground black pepper
1 cup chopped spinach
½ bell pepper, diced
1 slice sprouted grain bread
1 tablespoon hummus
¼ cup sauerkraut
½ cup cooked edamame

1. In a large nonstick skillet, cook the crumbled tofu over medium heat for 2 to 3 minutes until golden brown and crispy on the outside. Add the turmeric, salt, and pepper to taste and stir to combine. Add the spinach and bell pepper and cook for another 3 to 4 minutes until the vegetables soften.
2. Toast the bread and spread hummus on top.
3. Serve the tofu scramble with the sauerkraut, toast, and a side of edamame.

SERVING/STORAGE:
Tofu scramble keeps in the fridge for 3 to 4 days.
Store edamame in the fridge for up to 1 week.
Sauerkraut will keep for 1 to 2 months.

Tofu Scramble with Turmeric, Spinach, and Diced Tomatoes, Toast, and Sauerkraut

Another superfood plant-based breakfast scramble rich in flavor, probiotics, and veggie goodness. Even non-vegans are sure to swoon over this breakfast option.

Yield: 1 serving | Total Time: 10 minutes
Calories: 308 | Protein: 26g | Fiber: 9g

1 cup firm tofu, crumbled
1 teaspoon ground turmeric
1 cup chopped spinach
½ cup diced tomatoes
1 slice sprouted grain bread
¼ cup sauerkraut

1. In a large nonstick skillet, cook the crumbled tofu over medium heat for 2 to 3 minutes or until golden brown and crispy on the outside. Add the turmeric, spinach, and tomatoes, and cook for another 4 minutes until the vegetables soften.
2. Toast the sprouted grain bread to your liking.
3. Serve the tofu scramble with the toast and sauerkraut.

SERVING/STORAGE:
Best served fresh, especially the toast.
Tofu scramble can be stored in an airtight container in the fridge for 3 to 4 days.
After opening, sauerkraut keeps for for 1 to 2 months refrigerated.

Chia Pudding with Protein Powder, Blueberries, and Walnuts

A light vegan breakfast on the sweet side of delicious with tons of fiber to jump-start your metabolism for the day.

Yield: 1 serving | Total Time: ~10 minutes plus 2+ hours chilling time
Calories: 347 | Protein: 32g | Fiber: 16g

2 tablespoons chia seeds
½ cup almond milk
1 scoop plant-based protein powder
1 slice sprouted grain bread

¼ cup blueberries
1 tablespoon chopped walnuts

1. In a small bowl or jar, mix the chia seeds, almond milk, and protein powder. Stir well and refrigerate for at least 2 hours or overnight.
2. Toast the sprouted grain bread to your liking.
3. Top the chia pudding with blueberries and walnuts. Enjoy alongside the toast.

SERVING/STORAGE:

Chia pudding can be prepared ahead and stored in the fridge for up to 4 days.

Blueberries and walnuts can be added just before serving for freshness.

Protein Smoothie with Banana, Spinach, and Peanut Butter, Toast with Almond Butter, and Sauerkraut

In need of a quick-and-easy breakfast you can take with you in the morning? This vegan smoothie has everything you need to start your day with a clear mind and full belly.

Yield: 1 serving | Total Time: 10 minutes
Calories: 487 | Protein: 34g | Fiber: 9g

1 scoop plant-based protein powder
1 cup almond milk
½ banana
1 cup frozen spinach
1 tablespoon peanut butter
1 slice sprouted grain bread
1 tablespoon almond butter
½ cup sauerkraut

1. In a blender, combine the protein powder, almond milk, banana, spinach, and peanut butter until smooth.
2. Toast the sprouted grain bread and spread almond butter on top.
3. Serve the protein smoothie with toast and sauerkraut.

Smoothies are best served immediately but can be stored in the
fridge for up to 24 hours. Shake or stir before drinking if
separated.
After opening, sauerkraut keeps for 1 to 2 months in the fridge.

Tofu Scramble with Turmeric, Spinach, Mushrooms, Bell Peppers, and Avocado Toast

Start your day with a colorful and tasty tofu scramble. Fiber,
healthy fats, and lots of protein will make breakfast something
worth looking forward to.

Yield: 1 serving | Total Time: 15 minutes
Calories: 447 | Protein: 33g | Fiber: 17g

1 cup crumbled tofu
1 teaspoon ground turmeric
1 cup chopped spinach
½ cup sliced beech mushrooms
½ bell pepper, diced
1 slice sprouted grain bread
½ avocado, sliced
¼ cup sauerkraut

1. In a large nonstick skillet, cook the tofu over medium heat for 3
   to 4 minutes or until golden brown. Add the turmeric, spinach,
   mushrooms, and bell pepper. Cook for another 4 to 5 minutes until
   vegetables have softened.
2. Toast the sprouted grain bread and top with avocado slices.
3. Serve the tofu scramble with the avocado toast and sauerkraut.

SERVING/STORAGE:
Tofu scramble can be stored for up to 4 days in the fridge.
Avocado toast is best made fresh.
Sauerkraut keeps well for 1 to 2 months refrigerated.

Tofu Scramble with Spinach, Mushrooms, and Whole-Grain Toast with Vegan Yogurt

A light vegan breakfast scramble that will get you feeling energized and ready to tackle the day without worrying about what time lunch is.

Yield: 1 serving | Total Time: 12–15 minutes
Calories: 495 | Protein: 30g | Fiber: 9g

1 tablespoon extra-virgin olive oil
¼ cup sliced mushrooms
½ cup chopped spinach
½ block firm tofu, crumbled
Sea salt and ground black pepper
¼ cup nutritional yeast
1 slice whole-grain bread
½ cup unsweetened vegan yogurt (coconut- or almond-based)

1. In a large nonstick skillet, heat the olive oil over medium heat and sauté the mushrooms and spinach for 2 to 3 minutes or until tender. Add the tofu and cook, stirring occasionally, for 5 minutes until tofu is golden brown and crispy. Season with salt and pepper and sprinkle with nutritional yeast for a cheesy flavor.
2. Toast the whole-grain bread to your liking.
3. Scoop the vegan yogurt into a small dish on the side.

SERVING/STORAGE:
Tofu scramble can be stored up to 4 days and reheated. Toast and yogurt should be served fresh.

Peanut Butter Banana Smoothie with Hemp Protein and Oats

A delicious breakfast smoothie you can whip together in a pinch to get you where you need to go without skipping the most important meal of the day. It works great as a midday snack, too!

Yield: 1 serving | Total Time: 5 minutes
Calories: 490 | Protein: 30g | Fiber: 12g

- 1 frozen banana
- 1 tablespoon peanut butter
- ½ cup rolled oats
- 1 tablespoon hemp protein powder
- 1 cup unsweetened almond milk
- ¼ teaspoon ground cinnamon
- 1 tablespoon chia seeds

1. In a blender, combine the banana, peanut butter, oats, protein powder, almond milk, cinnamon, and chia seeds. Blend until smooth.
2. Pour the smoothie into a glass and enjoy!

SERVING/STORAGE:
Best consumed immediately.
Can refrigerate up to 24 hours (shake before drinking).

Omelet with Spinach, Mushrooms, and Edamame, with Sauerkraut

Classic omelet with a bit of a twist. This quick-and-easy breakfast is full of fresh foods, protein, fiber, and probiotics to feed your gut and your brain.

Yield: 1 serving | Total Time: 15 minutes
Calories: 455 | Protein: 30g | Fiber: 14g

- 1 teaspoon avocado oil
- 1 cup chopped spinach
- ½ cup sliced beech mushrooms

3 large eggs
½ cup edamame
¼ cup sauerkraut

1. In a large nonstick skillet, heat the oil over medium heat. Add the spinach and mushrooms and cook for 2 to 3 minutes until the spinach wilts and the mushrooms soften.
2. In a small bowl, whisk the eggs thoroughly and pour over the vegetables. Cook for 2 to 3 minutes until set and then fold into an omelet.
3. Serve the omelet with a side of edamame and sauerkraut.

SERVING/STORAGE:
   Best served fresh.
   Leftover omelet can be stored in the fridge for up to 2 days and
      reheated gently.
   Sauerkraut keeps for 1 to 2 months in the fridge.
   Edamame will keep for up to 1 week.

Protein Smoothie with Greek Yogurt, Spinach, Peanut Butter, and Sauerkraut

A probiotic protein smoothie with tons of flavor to get you focused for the day ahead.

Yield: 1 serving | Total Time: 5 minutes
Calories: 344 | Protein: 31g | Fiber: 7g

   1 scoop protein powder
   ½ cup Greek yogurt
   ½ banana
   1 cup frozen spinach
   1 tablespoon peanut butter
   ¼ cup sauerkraut

1. In a blender, combine the protein powder, Greek yogurt, banana, spinach, and peanut butter until smooth.
2. Serve the smoothie with sauerkraut on the side.

Best served immediately after blending.
Can store the smoothie in the fridge for up to 1 day (shake or
stir before drinking).
After opening, sauerkraut keeps for 1 to 2 months refrigerated.

Omelet with Spinach, Bell Peppers, Edamame, and Sauerkraut

A super delicious grain-free breakfast with just enough protein,
veggies, fiber, and probiotics to convince you that breakfast maybe
isn't so bad, right?

Yield: 1 serving | Total Time: ~15 minutes
Calories: 455 | Protein: 30g | Fiber: 15g

3 large eggs
1 cup chopped spinach
½ bell pepper, diced
½ cup edamame
¼ cup sauerkraut

1. In a large nonstick skillet, cook the spinach and bell pepper over
   medium heat for 2 to 3 minutes until softened.
2. In a small bowl, whisk the eggs until well combined and then pour
   over the vegetables. Cook for 2 to 3 minutes until set, then fold
   into an omelet.
3. Serve the omelet with a side of edamame and sauerkraut.

SERVING/STORAGE:
Best served immediately.
Omelet can be stored for up to 2 days refrigerated;
reheat gently.
Edamame and sauerkraut can be preportioned for convenience.

Omelet with Mushrooms, Spinach, Garlic, and Nutritional Yeast, with Avocado and Sauerkraut

A savory omelet with bold flavors and nutrient-dense ingredients that is so good, you won't even need to add salt.

Yield: 1 serving | Total Time: ~15 minutes
Calories: 451 | Protein: 30g | Fiber: 11g

> 1 teaspoon avocado oil
> 1 garlic clove, minced
> ½ cup sliced button mushrooms
> 1 cup chopped spinach
> 3 large eggs
> 2 tablespoons nutritional yeast
> ½ avocado, sliced
> ¼ cup sauerkraut

1. In a large nonstick skillet, heat the avocado oil over medium heat. Add the garlic and nutritional yeast and sauté for 1 minute. Add the mushrooms and spinach and cook for 3 to 4 minutes until softened.
2. In a small bowl, whisk the eggs thoroughly and then pour over the vegetables. Cook until set then fold into an omelet.
3. Serve the omelet with sliced avocado and sauerkraut on the side.

SERVING/STORAGE:
Best served fresh.
Omelet can be refrigerated for up to 2 days; reheat gently.

Scrambled Eggs with Sautéed Kale, Mushrooms, and Cherry Tomatoes, with Avocado and Sauerkraut

Grain-free and delicious! Not only is this super easy to make, but it tastes great and looks pretty on the plate. The camera eats first!

Yield: 1 serving | Total Time: ~15 minutes
Calories: 475 | Protein: 30g | Fiber: 10g

> 1 teaspoon avocado oil
> ½ cup sliced button mushrooms

1 cup chopped kale
½ cup cherry tomatoes, halved
3 large eggs
2 egg whites
½ avocado, sliced
¼ cup sauerkraut

1. In a large nonstick skillet, heat the oil over medium heat. Add the mushrooms, kale, and cherry tomatoes, and cook for 3 to 4 minutes until tender.
2. In a small bowl, whisk the eggs and egg whites and pour over the vegetables. Scramble for 2 to 3 minutes until cooked through.
3. Serve the scrambled eggs with sliced avocado and sauerkraut.

SERVING/STORAGE:
Best served immediately.
Store leftover eggs in the fridge for up to 4 days, but the texture may change upon reheating.

Scrambled Eggs with Spinach, Mushrooms, and Avocado

A simple yet highly effective breakfast with everything you need to kick-start your morning.

Yield: 1 serving | Total Time: 10 minutes
Calories: 495 | Protein: 30g | Fiber: 9g

1 tablespoon extra-virgin olive oil
¼ cup sliced button mushrooms
½ cup chopped spinach
3 large eggs
Sea salt and ground black pepper
¼ cup shredded cheddar cheese (optional)
½ avocado, sliced

1. In a large nonstick skillet, heat the olive oil over medium heat and cook the mushrooms and spinach for 2 to 3 minutes until tender. Crack the eggs into the pan and scramble, adding salt and pepper, then cook for 2 to 3 minutes until fully set. Add the cheese (if desired).

2. Plate the scrambled eggs and top with sliced avocado.

SERVING/STORAGE:

Best fresh.

Scrambled eggs can be stored for up to 4 days; reheat gently.

Avocado should be sliced just before serving.

Scrambled Eggs with Sautéed Spinach, Cherry Tomatoes, and Bacon

This one can be made with or without bacon depending on your dietary preferences. Either way, it's a tasty breakfast where you'll find yourself going back for seconds.

Yield: 1 serving | Total Time: 10–12 minutes
Calories: 490 | Protein: 30g | Fiber: 6g

  1 teaspoon extra-virgin olive oil
  1 cup chopped spinach
  3 large eggs
  Sea salt and ground black pepper
  2 slices cooked bacon, crumbled
  5–6 cherry tomatoes, halved

1. In a large nonstick skillet, heat the olive oil over medium heat and sauté the spinach for 1 to 2 minutes until wilted. Add the eggs, salt, and pepper and scramble until fully cooked.
2. Stir in the bacon and tomatoes just before finishing.

SERVING/STORAGE:

Best fresh.

Cooked eggs and bacon can be stored for up to 4 days in the fridge.

Tomatoes should be added fresh.

LUNCH

Grilled Chicken Salad with Avocado, Quinoa, and Kimchi

A protein-packed midday meal with tons of fiber—add your favorite spices or dressings for an added flavor boost!

Yield: 1 serving | Total Time: 20–25 minutes
Calories: 530 | Protein: 40g | Fiber: 10g

For the Chicken

> 4-ounce boneless, skinless chicken breast
> 2 teaspoons extra-virgin olive oil
> Sea salt and ground black pepper

For the Salad

> 3 cups mixed greens (e.g., spinach, arugula, romaine)
> ½ avocado, sliced
> ½ cucumber, sliced
> ½ cup shredded carrots
> 1 tablespoon extra-virgin olive oil
> 1 tablespoon lemon juice
>
> ½ cup cooked quinoa
> ½ cup kimchi

1. For the chicken: Preheat your grill or grill pan over medium-high heat. Rub the chicken breast with the olive oil and season with salt and pepper. Grill the chicken for about 6 to 7 minutes per side, or until the internal temperature reaches 165°F and the chicken is fully cooked. Once cooked, let the chicken rest for a few minutes before slicing into thin strips.
2. For the salad: While the chicken is grilling, place the mixed greens in a large bowl. Add the avocado, cucumber, and carrots to the salad.

3. For the dressing: In a small bowl, whisk together the olive oil and lemon juice until well combined. Season with a pinch of salt and pepper, if desired.
4. Assemble the salad: Place the grilled chicken strips on top of the mixed greens salad. Drizzle the olive oil and lemon dressing over the salad and toss gently to coat.
5. For serving: Serve the salad with the quinoa on the side. Add a serving of kimchi to the plate to complete the meal.

SERVING/STORAGE:
Best enjoyed fresh.
Grilled chicken can be stored in the fridge for up to 3 days.
Quinoa and chopped veggies can be prepped in advance and
    kept refrigerated for 2 to 3 days.
Avocado and dressing should be added just before serving.
Once opened, kimchi stays fresh in the fridge for up to
    3 months.

Grilled Chicken Breast with Roasted Sweet Potato and Green Beans, Salad with Kimchi

A hearty lunch with protein and veggies to keep your mind sharp and stomach full all the way through to dinnertime.

Yield: 1 serving | Total Time: 25–30 minutes
Calories: 445 | Protein: 37g | Fiber: 9g

For the Chicken

    4-ounce boneless, skinless chicken breast
    Sea salt and ground black pepper
    Extra-virgin olive oil

For the Sweet Potato and Green Beans

    1 medium sweet potato, cut into cubes
    ½ cup green beans, trimmed
    2 teaspoons extra-virgin olive oil
    Sea salt and ground black pepper

For the Salad

    3 cups spinach
    ½ cucumber, sliced
    ½ cup shredded carrots
    1 tablespoon extra-virgin olive oil
    1 tablespoon lemon juice

    ½ cup kimchi

1. For the chicken: Preheat your grill or grill pan over medium-high heat. Season the chicken with salt, pepper, and a little olive oil. Grill the chicken for 6 to 7 minutes per side, or until fully cooked (165°F internal temperature).
2. For the sweet potato and green beans: Preheat the oven to 400°F (200°C). Toss the cubed sweet potato and green beans with 2 teaspoons olive oil, salt, and pepper. Spread them out on a baking sheet and roast for 20 to 25 minutes, flipping halfway, until the sweet potato is tender and the green beans are cooked.
3. For the salad: In a large bowl, combine the spinach, cucumber slices, and carrots. For the dressing, whisk together the olive oil and lemon juice. Drizzle over the salad and toss to combine.
4. For serving: Serve the grilled chicken with the roasted sweet potatoes, green beans, and the fresh salad. Add a serving of kimchi on the side to complete the meal.

SERVING/STORAGE:
    Chicken and roasted veggies can be stored in the fridge for up to 3 days.
    Salad is best fresh; dressing can be stored separately for 2 to 3 days.
    Kimchi stores well for up to 3 months once opened.

Turkey and Avocado Wrap with Roasted Cauliflower and Kimchi

The perfect packed lunch with bold flavors and hearty ingredients. Your coworker might just try to steal this one from the communal fridge if you aren't careful.

Yield: 1 serving | Total Time: 25–30 minutes
Calories: 365 | Protein: 27g | Fiber: 10g

1 whole-grain tortilla
4 ounces sliced turkey breast
½ avocado, sliced
1 cup mixed greens (e.g., spinach, lettuce, arugula)
1 tablespoon mustard of choice

½ small cauliflower, cut into florets
1 tablespoon extra-virgin olive oil
Sea salt and ground black pepper

¼ cup kimchi

1. Lay the whole-grain tortilla flat on a clean surface. Layer the turkey slices, avocado, mixed greens, and mustard on the tortilla. Roll the tortilla up tightly and slice it in half.
2. Preheat the oven to 400°F (200°C). Toss the cauliflower florets with the olive oil and season with salt and pepper. Spread them out on a baking sheet and roast for 20 to 25 minutes, flipping halfway, until crispy and tender.
3. Serve the turkey and avocado wrap with the roasted cauliflower on the side along with a serving of kimchi.

SERVING/STORAGE:
The wrap can be assembled ahead of time (without the avocado) and stored for 1 day.
Roasted cauliflower keeps in the fridge for 2 to 3 days.
Kimchi stores well for up to 3 months after opening.

Grilled Chicken Salad with Quinoa and Kimchi

A light lunch packed with protein, guaranteed to satisfy your cravings.

Yield: 1 serving | Total Time: 25–30 minutes
Calories: 450 | Protein: 39g | Fiber: 7g

For the Chicken

> 4-ounce boneless, skinless chicken breast
> 1 tablespoon extra-virgin olive oil
> Sea salt and ground black pepper

For the Salad

> 2 cups mixed greens (e.g., spinach, arugula, romaine)
> ½ cup shredded carrots
> ½ cup sliced cucumbers
> Extra virgin olive oil
> 1 tablespoon lemon juice
>
> ½ cup cooked quinoa
> ½ cup kimchi

1. For the chicken: Preheat your grill or grill pan over medium-high heat. Rub the chicken breast with the olive oil and season with salt and pepper. Grill the chicken for 6 to 7 minutes per side or until the internal temperature reaches 165°F.
2. For the salad: In a large bowl, toss the mixed greens, shredded carrots, and cucumber slices. Drizzle with olive oil and lemon juice and toss to coat.
3. Slice the grilled chicken and place it on top of the salad.
4. Serve the quinoa on the side along with a serving of kimchi.

SERVING/STORAGE:
> The salad and chicken are best served fresh.
> The chicken can be stored up to 4 days refrigerated.
> Kimchi stored in the fridge will last for up to 3 months.
> Quinoa can be stored in the fridge for 3 to 4 days.

Grilled Turkey Burger with Roasted Sweet Potato, Steamed Broccoli, and Salad with Kimchi

A hearty low-fat lunch with tons of veggies—perfect for the family or for meal prep.

Yield: 1 serving | Total Time: 30 minutes
Calories: 432 | Protein: 32g | Fiber: 9g

For the Burger

> 4 ounces ground turkey
> Sea salt and ground black pepper
> ½ teaspoon extra-virgin olive oil

For the Sweet Potato

> 1 medium sweet potato, cubed
> Extra-virgin olive oil
> Salt and pepper

For the Broccoli

> 1 cup broccoli florets

For the Salad

> 2 cups mixed greens (e.g., spinach, arugula, romaine)
> ½ cucumber, sliced
> ½ cup shredded cabbage
> 1 tablespoon extra-virgin olive oil
> 1 tablespoon lemon juice

> ½ cup kimchi

1. For the burger: Preheat a grill or grill pan over medium heat. Season the ground turkey with salt, pepper, and a little olive oil and form into a patty. Grill the turkey burger for 5 to 6 minutes per side, or until it reaches an internal temperature of 165°F.
2. For the sweet potato: Preheat the oven to 400°F (200°C). Toss the sweet potato cubes with a little olive oil, salt, and pepper. Spread them out on a baking sheet and roast for 20 to 25 minutes, flipping halfway, until the sweet potatoes are tender.

3. For the broccoli: While the turkey and sweet potatoes cook, add a tablespoon of water to a saucepan and steam the broccoli florets on medium heat for about 4 to 5 minutes or until tender.
4. For the salad: In a large bowl, combine the mixed greens, cucumber, and shredded cabbage. For the dressing, whisk together the olive oil and lemon juice. Drizzle over the salad and toss to combine.
5. Serve the grilled turkey burger with the roasted sweet potato, steamed broccoli, salad, and kimchi.

SERVING/STORAGE:
Store the turkey burger in the fridge for up to 3 days.
Store the roasted sweet potato for up to 5 days in the fridge.
Store the steamed broccoli for 2 to 3 days.
Keep the salad ingredients separate and assemble fresh.
Kimchi will last for up to 3 months in the fridge.

Turkey Lettuce Wraps with Hummus, Quinoa, and Sauerkraut

Deceptively filling, with flavors that will have even your kids finishing their plate. Don't sleep on this protein-rich, low-carb, healthy lunch option.

Yield: 1 serving | Total Time: 10 minutes
Calories: 520 | Protein: 35g | Fiber: 9g

2 large lettuce leaves
¼ cup hummus
4 ounces lean turkey breast, sliced
¼ cucumber, sliced
½ cup cooked quinoa
¼ cup sauerkraut
1 tablespoon extra-virgin olive oil
Sea salt and ground black pepper

1. Lay the lettuce leaves flat and spread a thin layer of hummus on each. Place the turkey slices on top followed by the cucumber slices. Wrap the lettuce around the filling to create wraps.

2. Place the cooked quinoa on the side.
3. Add the sauerkraut on the side as a probiotic option. Drizzle with olive oil and season with salt and pepper.

SERVING/STORAGE:
Best fresh.
Can refrigerate the components separately for up to 2 days.
Assemble the wraps just before eating.

Tuna Salad with Avocado, Chickpeas, and Kimchi

A tasty twist on classic tuna salad with plenty of protein and fiber to keep you satisfied and sharp throughout the day.

Yield: 1 serving | Total Time: 8 minutes
Calories: 530 | Protein: 35g | Fiber: 13g

4 ounces canned tuna in water, drained
½ avocado, diced
¼ cup cooked chickpeas
¼ cup chopped cucumber
1 tablespoon extra-virgin olive oil
1 tablespoon lemon juice
½ cup kimchi

1. In a bowl, combine the tuna, avocado, chickpeas, and cucumber.
2. In a separate bowl, whisk together the olive oil and lemon juice. Pour over the tuna salad and toss gently.
3. Add the kimchi as a side for probiotics.

SERVING/STORAGE:
Enjoy fresh or store salad (without avocado) for up to 1 day.
Add fresh avocado and kimchi before serving.

Lentil and Vegetable Stew with Side Salad and Kimchi

I'm a sucker for a good stew, and this is a go-to of mine. It's the perfect meal-prep recipe, especially during the wintertime.

Yield: 1 serving | Total Time: 20–25 minutes
Calories: 369 | Protein: 23g | Fiber: 21g

For the Stew

    1 medium carrot, chopped
    2 celery stalks, chopped
    1 cup fresh or canned diced tomatoes
    1 cup cooked lentils
    3 tablespoons vegetable broth

For the Salad

    3 cups mixed greens (e.g., spinach, arugula, romaine)
    ½ cup shredded cabbage
    1 tablespoon hemp seeds
    1 tablespoon tahini
    1 tablespoon lemon juice

    ½ cup kimchi

1. In a large pot, cook the carrots, celery, and tomatoes over medium heat for 5 minutes until tender. Add the cooked lentils and 3 tablespoons of vegetable broth and simmer for 10 minutes, allowing the flavors to combine.
2. In a bowl, mix the greens, shredded cabbage, and hemp seeds. Dress with tahini and lemon juice.
3. Serve the lentil stew with the salad and a side of kimchi.

SERVING/STORAGE:
    Stew can be refrigerated for 4 to 5 days or frozen up to 2 months.
    Salad is best assembled fresh; keep dressing separate until ready to eat.
    Kimchi keeps for up to 3 months in the fridge.

Lentil and Chickpea Salad with Sweet Potato Wedges and Kimchi

A yummy vegan salad option rich in fiber and flavor. Sprinkle with nutritional yeast for an extra bit of flavor.

Yield: 1 serving | Total Time: 30 minutes
Calories: 492 | Protein: 19g | Fiber: 19g

For the Salad

½ cup cooked lentils
½ cup cooked chickpeas
½ cucumber, diced
½ cup cherry tomatoes, halved
1 tablespoon extra-virgin olive oil
1 tablespoon lemon juice

For the Sweet Potato

1 medium sweet potato, cut into wedges
Extra-virgin olive oil
Salt and pepper

½ cup kimchi

1. For the salad: In a medium bowl, combine the lentils, chickpeas, cucumber, and cherry tomatoes. Dress with olive oil and lemon juice.
2. For the sweet potato wedges: Preheat the oven to 400°F (200°C). Toss the sweet potato wedges with olive oil, salt, and pepper. Spread them out on a baking sheet and roast for 25 minutes, flipping halfway, until desired tenderness.
3. Serve the salad with the roasted sweet potato wedges and kimchi.

SERVING/STORAGE:
Salad can be stored in the fridge for up to 2 days (keep dressing separate if meal prepping).
Roasted sweet potatoes can be stored in the fridge for up to 5 days.
Kimchi keeps for up to 3 months when refrigerated properly.

Vegan Chickpea Wrap with Roasted Brussels Sprouts and Kimchi

A wrap so tasty your non-vegan friends won't even notice there isn't any meat. This is one of my favorite plant-based lunches that stays in my rotation for a reason.

Yield: 1 serving | Total Time: ~30 minutes
Calories: 412 | Protein: 17g | Fiber: 18g

For the Wrap

> 1 whole-grain tortilla
> ½ cup cooked chickpeas
> ½ avocado, sliced
> ¼ cup shredded carrots

For the Sprouts

> 1 cup roasted Brussels sprouts
> Extra-virgin olive oil
> Sea salt and ground black pepper

> ¼ cup kimchi

1. For the chickpea wrap: In a nonstick skillet or in the microwave, warm the tortilla slightly. In the center of the tortilla, layer the chickpeas, avocado, and carrots. Roll up the tortilla to form a wrap.
2. For the Brussels sprouts: Preheat the oven to 400°F (200°C). Toss the Brussels sprouts with olive oil, salt, and pepper. Spread them out on a baking sheet and roast for 20 to 25 minutes, flipping halfway, until crispy.
3. Serve the chickpea wrap with a side of roasted Brussels sprouts and kimchi.

SERVING/STORAGE:
> The wrap is best fresh but can be stored wrapped in foil or parchment for 1 day.
> Roasted Brussels sprouts keep for up to 5 days in the fridge.
> Kimchi lasts for up to 3 months when stored refrigerated in a sealed container.

Lentil and Chickpea Salad with Roasted Sweet Potato and Kimchi

A light and flavorful salad option full of fiber. This salad alone gets you the majority of your daily recommended fiber intake.

Yield: 1 serving | Total Time: 30–35 minutes
Calories: 477 | Protein: 23g | Fiber: 23g

For the Salad

> ½ cup cooked lentils
> ½ cup cooked chickpeas
> 1 cup shredded kale
> ½ cucumber, diced
> ½ cup cherry tomatoes, halved
> 1 tablespoon tahini
> 1 tablespoon lemon juice

For the Sweet Potato

> 1 medium sweet potato, cut into wedges
> Extra-virgin olive oil
> Sea salt and ground black pepper

> ½ cup kimchi

1. For the salad: In a large bowl, combine the lentils, chickpeas, kale, cucumber, and cherry tomatoes. Dress with tahini and lemon juice.
2. For the sweet potato wedges: Preheat the oven to 400°F (200°C). Toss the sweet potato wedges with olive oil, salt, and pepper. Spread them out on a baking sheet and roast for 25 minutes until desired tenderness.
3. Serve the lentil and chickpea salad with the roasted sweet potato wedges and kimchi.

SERVING/STORAGE:
Salad ingredients can be prepped and stored separately for 2 to 3 days.
Roasted sweet potatoes last up to 5 days refrigerated.
Kimchi keeps well for up to 3 months in a sealed container.

Quinoa Bowl with Roasted Chickpeas, Cabbage, Kale, and Tahini Dressing

My version of a Mediterranean bowl that's plant-based and high in both protein and fiber.

Yield: 1 serving | Total Time: ~30 minutes
Calories: 433 | Protein: 21g | Fiber: 19g

For the Quinoa

    ½ cup cooked quinoa
    ½ cup roasted chickpeas
    ½ cup shredded cabbage
    ½ cup chopped kale
    1 tablespoon tahini dressing

For the Brussels Sprouts

    1 cup roasted Brussels sprouts
    Extra-virgin olive oil
    Sea salt and ground black pepper

    ½ cup kimchi

1. In a bowl, combine the quinoa, chickpeas, cabbage, and kale. Drizzle with tahini dressing.
2. Preheat the oven to 400°F (200°C). Toss the Brussels sprouts with olive oil, salt, and pepper. Spread them out on a baking sheet and roast for 20 to 25 minutes until desired tenderness.
3. Serve the quinoa bowl with roasted Brussels sprouts and kimchi.

SERVING/STORAGE:
    Bowl ingredients can be stored separately in the fridge for 3 to 4 days.
    Tahini dressing can be prepped in bulk and stored up to a week.
    Kimchi stays fresh in the fridge for up to 3 months.

Chickpea Salad with Avocado, Cucumber, and Kimchi

This light and refreshing salad is perfect as a meal or a side dish—either way, it's delicious and a healthy addition to any menu.

Yield: 1 serving | Total Time: 8–10 minutes
Calories: 510 | Protein: 15g | Fiber: 13g

½ cup canned chickpeas, drained and rinsed
½ avocado, diced
¼ cucumber, sliced
¼ cup thinly sliced red onion
1 tablespoon extra-virgin olive oil
1 tablespoon lemon juice

½ cup kimchi

1. In a medium bowl, combine the chickpeas, avocado, cucumber, and onion.
2. In a small bowl, whisk together the olive oil and lemon juice. Pour over the salad and toss gently.
3. Add kimchi on the side for probiotics.

SERVING/STORAGE:
Store salad (without avocado) for up to 1 day.
Add avocado and kimchi fresh before serving.

Lentil Salad with Roasted Veggies and Tahini Dressing

I love a good lentil salad, and this one is perfect for meal prep. With access to preroasted veggies, this salad can be thrown together in no time.

Yield: 1 serving | Total Time: 10 minutes (if veggies are preroasted)
Calories: 520 | Protein: 28g | Fiber: 14g

½ cup cooked lentils
½ cup roasted cauliflower
½ cup roasted carrots
1 tablespoon tahini
1 tablespoon lemon juice

1 tablespoon extra-virgin olive oil
Sea salt
1 tablespoon chopped fresh parsley

1. In a large bowl, combine the lentils, cauliflower, and carrots.
2. In a small bowl, whisk together the tahini, lemon juice, olive oil, and a pinch of salt. Drizzle over the salad and toss to coat.
3. Sprinkle chopped parsley over the salad.

SERVING/STORAGE:
   Store assembled salad (minus dressing) for up to 2 days.
   Add dressing and parsley just before serving.

Grilled Chicken Thigh with Side Salad and Kimchi

A low-calorie, high-protein, and grain-free lunch option that works just as well for dinner!

Yield: 1 serving | Total Time: 20–25 minutes
Calories: 489 | Protein: 33g | Fiber: 8g

   4-ounce chicken thigh

For the Salad

   3 cups mixed greens (e.g., spinach, arugula, romaine)
   ½ cup shredded carrots
   ½ cucumber, sliced
   ½ red bell pepper, sliced
   2 tablespoons sunflower seeds
   1 tablespoon extra-virgin olive oil
   1 tablespoon lemon juice

   ¼ cup kimchi

1. On a nonstick skillet at medium heat, cook the chicken thigh for about 6 to 7 minutes per side or until fully cooked (internal temperature of 165°F).
2. In a large bowl, toss the mixed greens, carrots, cucumber, bell pepper, and sunflower seeds. Drizzle with olive oil and lemon juice.
3. Serve the grilled chicken thigh with the side salad and kimchi.

Chicken and salad can be refrigerated separately for
2 to 3 days.

Add the dressing just before eating.

Kimchi keeps in the fridge for up to 3 months.

Grilled Shrimp with Mashed Cauliflower, Roasted Zucchini, and Mixed Greens Salad

For fans of seafood, this grilled shrimp lunch is the perfect low-calorie midday meal to keep you going. Lunch doesn't have to be boring!

Yield: 1 serving | Total Time: 25–30 minutes
Calories: 319 | Protein: 30g | Fiber: 7g

4 ounces shrimp, peeled and deveined

For the Zucchini

1 medium zucchini, sliced
Extra-virgin olive oil
Sea salt

For the Cauliflower

1 cup cauliflower florets

For the Salad

3 cups mixed greens (e.g., spinach, arugula, romaine)
½ cup shredded carrots
1 tablespoon extra-virgin olive oil
1 tablespoon lemon juice

½ cup kimchi

1. For the shrimp: Grill shrimp on medium-high heat for 2 to 3 minutes per side or until opaque and cooked through.
2. For the zucchini: Preheat the oven to 400°F (200°C). Toss the zucchini slices with olive oil and salt. Spread them out on a baking sheet and roast for 15 minutes.

3. For the cauliflower: Add a tablespoon of water to a saucepan and steam the cauliflower florets on medium heat for about 10 minutes until tender, then mash with a fork or potato masher.
4. For the salad: Toss the mixed greens with the carrots. Dress with olive oil and lemon juice.
5. Serve the grilled shrimp with mashed cauliflower, roasted zucchini, salad, and a side of kimchi.

SERVING/STORAGE:
Shrimp is best fresh but can be refrigerated for up to 2 days.
Mashed cauliflower and roasted zucchini keep for 2 to 3 days refrigerated.
Salad is best undressed if prepping ahead.
Kimchi keeps for up to 3 months in the fridge.

Grilled Turkey Burger with Mashed Cauliflower, Green Beans, and Salad with Kimchi

Hearty yet low-calorie, this turkey burger is perfect for days when you feel like lunch just can't come soon enough.

Yield: 1 serving | Total Time: ~30 minutes
Calories: 370 | Protein: 33g | Fiber: 9g

4-ounce turkey burger patty
1 cup cauliflower florets
½ cup green beans, trimmed
3 cups mixed greens (e.g., spinach, arugula, romaine)
½ cup shredded cabbage
1 tablespoon extra-virgin olive oil
1 tablespoon lemon juice

½ cup kimchi

1. Preheat a grill or grill pan over medium heat. Grill the turkey patty for about 5 to 6 minutes per side or until it reaches an internal temperature of 165°F.
2. Steam the cauliflower florets for about 10 minutes until tender. Mash with a fork or potato masher.

3. Steam the green beans for 4 to 5 minutes or until tender but still bright green.
4. In a large bowl, toss the mixed greens and shredded cabbage with olive oil and lemon juice.
5. Serve the grilled turkey burger with mashed cauliflower, steamed green beans, salad, and a side of kimchi.

SERVING/STORAGE:
    Turkey burger, mashed cauliflower, and green beans can be prepped and stored for 3 days in the fridge.
    Dress the salad just before eating.
    Kimchi keeps well for up to 3 months refrigerated.

Grilled Chicken Thigh with Roasted Brussels Sprouts, Mashed Rutabaga, Salad, and Kimchi

High in protein and packed with veggies, this is a great option that's not too much, not too little, just right.

Yield: 1 serving | Total Time: ~35 minutes
Calories: 474 | Protein: 35g | Fiber: 13g

For the Chicken

    4-ounce chicken thigh

For the Brussels Sprouts

    1 cup halved Brussels sprouts
    Extra-virgin olive oil
    Sea salt and ground black pepper

For the Rutabaga

    1 medium rutabaga, peeled and cubed

For the Salad

    3 cups mixed greens (e.g., spinach, arugula, romaine)
    ½ cup shredded carrots

1 tablespoon extra-virgin olive oil
1 tablespoon lemon juice

½ cup kimchi

1. For the chicken: Grill the chicken thigh on medium-high heat for 6 to 7 minutes per side or until fully cooked (165°F internal temperature).
2. For the Brussels sprouts: Preheat the oven to 400°F (200°C). Toss the Brussels sprouts with olive oil, salt, and pepper. Spread them out on a baking sheet and roast for 20 to 25 minutes until tender and slightly browned.
3. For the rutabaga: In a medium saucepan over medium heat, boil the rutabaga cubes for 15 to 20 minutes until tender. Use enough water so that the cubes are fully submerged throughout. Mash with a fork or potato masher.
4. For the salad: Toss the mixed greens and carrots with the olive oil and lemon juice.
5. Serve the grilled chicken thigh with roasted Brussels sprouts, mashed rutabaga, salad, and kimchi.

SERVING/STORAGE:
Chicken and sides can be prepped 3 to 4 days ahead and refrigerated.
Store the salad and kimchi separately in the refrigerator to keep fresh.

Grilled Chicken Breast with Roasted Zucchini, Steamed Broccoli, Salad, and Kimchi

This meal is low-calorie, though you wouldn't know it based on how delicious it is. It's a decadent lunch fit for a queen.

Yield: 1 serving | Total Time: ~30 minutes
Calories: 365 | Protein: 35g | Fiber: 11g

For the Chicken

4-ounce boneless, skinless chicken breast

For the Zucchini

> 1 medium zucchini, sliced
> Extra-virgin olive oil
> Sea salt

For the Broccoli

> 1 cup broccoli florets

For the Salad

> 3 cups mixed greens (e.g., spinach, arugula, romaine)
> ½ cup shredded carrots
> 1 tablespoon extra-virgin olive oil
> 1 tablespoon lemon juice

> ½ cup kimchi

1. For the chicken: Grill the chicken breast on medium heat for about 6 to 7 minutes per side or until fully cooked (165°F internal temperature).
2. For the zucchini: Preheat the oven to 400°F (200°C). Toss the zucchini with olive oil and salt. Spread them out on a baking sheet and roast for 15 minutes or until tender.
3. For the broccoli: Steam the broccoli for 4 to 5 minutes or until bright green and tender.
4. For the salad: Toss the mixed greens with the carrots. Dress the salad with olive oil and lemon juice.
5. Serve the grilled chicken breast with roasted zucchini, steamed broccoli, salad, and kimchi.

SERVING/STORAGE:
The chicken, zucchini, and broccoli can be stored in the fridge for 2 to 3 days.
Keep the salad and kimchi separate to maintain freshness.

Grilled Chicken Salad with Avocado, Cucumber, and Kimchi

For fans of chicken salad, add this recipe to your rotation ASAP. You could even make this into a wrap or sandwich if that's your vibe.

Yield: 1 serving | Total Time: 15–20 minutes
Calories: 510 | Protein: 40 | Fiber:13g

For the Chicken

> 4-ounce boneless, skinless chicken breast
> 1 tablespoon extra-virgin olive oil
> Sea salt and ground black pepper

For the Salad

> 2 cups mixed greens (e.g., spinach, arugula, romaine)
> ½ avocado, sliced
> ¼ cucumber, sliced
> ¼ cup shredded carrots
> 1 tablespoon extra-virgin olive oil
> 1 tablespoon lemon juice

> ½ cup kimchi

1. For the chicken: Preheat a grill or grill pan to medium-high heat. Rub the chicken with olive oil and season with salt and pepper. Grill for about 6 to 7 minutes per side until cooked through (165°F internal temperature). Slice thinly.
2. For the salad: In a large bowl, combine the mixed greens, avocado, cucumber, and carrots. Whisk together the olive oil and lemon juice. Drizzle over the salad and toss.
3. Add kimchi on the side for probiotics.

SERVING/STORAGE:
> Store the salad (without dressing or avocado) for up to 2 days in the refrigerator.
> Add the dressing and avocado fresh.
> The chicken can be grilled ahead and chilled.

Turkey Lettuce Wraps with Avocado, Cucumber, and Kimchi

Like a turkey sandwich but better. This turkey wrap is light, refreshing, and packed with protein.

Yield: 1 serving | Total Time: 5–7 minutes
Calories: 430 | Protein: 38g | Fiber: 10g

  4 ounces cooked turkey breast, sliced
  1 large lettuce leaf (romaine or butter lettuce)
  ½ avocado, sliced
  ¼ cucumber, sliced
  ¼ cup kimchi

1. Lay the turkey slices in the lettuce leaf and top with the avocado and cucumber.
2. Add kimchi on the side for probiotics.

SERVING/STORAGE:
  Assemble fresh.
  Turkey and veggies can be prepped in advance and stored for 2 to 3 days.

DINNER

Grilled Salmon with Roasted Brussels Sprouts, Sweet Potato Wedges, Lentils, and Steamed Asparagus

Protein-packed and so good you'll think it was from a restaurant. This is a recipe your family will want again and again.

Yield: 1 serving | Total Time: 30–35 minutes
Calories: 531 | Protein: 40g | Fiber: 40g

For the Salmon

  4-ounce salmon fillet
  1 teaspoon extra-virgin olive oil
  Sea salt and ground black pepper

For the Sprouts and Wedges

½ cup Brussels sprouts, trimmed and halved
½ medium sweet potato, cut into wedges
1 teaspoon extra-virgin olive oil
Sea salt and ground black pepper

For the Lentils

½ cup cooked lentils

For the Asparagus

½ cup chopped asparagus stalks
Lemon wedge (optional)

1. For the salmon: Preheat your grill or grill pan over medium-high heat. Rub the salmon with olive oil and season with salt and pepper. Grill the salmon for about 4 to 5 minutes per side or until it reaches an internal temperature of 145°F and flakes easily with a fork. Set aside.
2. For the Brussels sprouts and sweet potato wedges: Preheat the oven to 400°F (200°C). Toss the Brussels sprouts and sweet potato wedges in 1 teaspoon olive oil and season with salt and pepper. Spread them out on a baking sheet and roast for 20 to 25 minutes, flipping halfway through, until the Brussels sprouts are crispy and the sweet potatoes are tender.
3. For the lentils: If not already cooked, prepare the lentils according to package instructions.
4. For the asparagus: While the vegetables roast, add a tablespoon of water to a saucepan and steam the asparagus on medium heat for about 4 to 5 minutes or until tender but still vibrant green.
5. Serve the grilled salmon alongside the Brussels sprouts and sweet potato wedges. Add the cooked lentils and steamed asparagus to complete the meal. Optionally, squeeze a wedge of lemon over the salmon for added flavor.

SERVING/STORAGE:
Best served hot and fresh.

Cooked salmon can be stored in the fridge for up to 4 days and
reheated gently.

Roasted veggies and lentils can be prepped in advance and
stored for 3 to 4 days in the fridge.

Asparagus is best when fresh but can be stored for up to 5 days
in the fridge.

Lemon, if using, should be added just before serving.

Baked Salmon with Steamed Broccoli, Quinoa, and Roasted Brussels Sprouts

This is a low-calorie dinner perfect for days when you ate a big lunch
but still want to make sure you're getting your 30–30–3 in for the day.

Yield: 1 serving | Total Time: 30 minutes
Calories: 444 | Protein: 33g | Fiber: 9g

For the Salmon

> 4-ounce salmon fillet
> 1 teaspoon extra-virgin olive oil
> Sea salt and ground black pepper

For the Broccoli

> ½ cup broccoli florets

For the Brussels Sprouts

> ½ cup halved Brussels sprouts
> 1 teaspoon extra-virgin olive oil
> Sea salt and ground black pepper

> ½ cup cooked quinoa

1. For the salmon: Preheat the oven to 400°F (200°C). Rub the
   salmon fillet with 1 teaspoon olive oil and season with salt and
   pepper. Place the salmon on a baking sheet and bake for 12 to 15
   minutes or until the salmon flakes easily with a fork.
2. For the broccoli: While the salmon bakes, steam the broccoli
   florets for about 5 to 7 minutes until tender but still vibrant green.

3. For the Brussels sprouts: Toss the halved Brussels sprouts with 1 teaspoon olive oil, salt, and pepper. Spread them on a baking sheet and roast in the oven for 15 to 20 minutes, flipping halfway through, until crispy and golden brown.
4. If not already cooked, prepare the quinoa according to package instructions.
5. Serve the baked salmon alongside the steamed broccoli, quinoa, and roasted Brussels sprouts for a delicious, nutrient-packed dinner.

SERVING/STORAGE:
Salmon, quinoa, and veggies can be stored in the fridge for 3 to 4 days.
Best when served warm.
Brussels sprouts may lose crispness when stored—reheat in the oven for best results.

Grilled Shrimp with Zucchini Noodles, Cherry Tomatoes, Garlic, and Mixed Green Salad, with Sauerkraut

Not-your-average pasta dish. It's low-calorie, low-carb, and oh-so delicious.

Yield: 1 serving | Total Time: 20–25 minutes
Calories: 178 | Protein: 28g | Fiber: 5g

For the Shrimp

4 ounces shrimp, peeled and deveined
1 teaspoon extra-virgin olive oil
Sea salt and ground black pepper

For the Zucchini

1 teaspoon extra-virgin olive oil
1 garlic clove, minced
2 medium zucchini, spiralized into noodles
Salt and pepper

For the Salad

> 2 cups mixed greens (e.g., spinach, lettuce, arugula)
> ¼ cup sauerkraut
> ½ cup halved cherry tomatoes

1. For the shrimp: Preheat your grill or grill pan over medium heat. Toss the shrimp with the olive oil and season with salt and pepper. Grill the shrimp for 2 to 3 minutes per side until cooked through.
2. For the zucchini noodles: In a large nonstick skillet, heat 1 teaspoon olive oil over medium heat. Add the minced garlic and sauté for 1 minute. Add the zucchini noodles and sauté for 2 to 3 minutes until tender but still slightly crisp. Season with salt and pepper.
3. For the salad: In a medium bowl, place the mixed greens and top with the sauerkraut.
4. Serve the grilled shrimp on top of the zucchini noodles with cherry tomatoes. Enjoy with the side salad of mixed greens and sauerkraut.

SERVING/STORAGE:
Shrimp is best fresh but can be stored for up to 2 days.
Zucchini noodles are best when freshly cooked.
Salad and sauerkraut can be prepped ahead.

Baked Salmon with Roasted Brussels Sprouts, Mashed Sweet Potato, and Steamed Green Beans

Perfect for autumn, this is a great dinner option that is super healthy and sure to impress your dinner guests.

Yield: 1 serving | Total Time: ~35 minutes
Calories: 416 | Protein: 30g | Fiber: 9g

For the Salmon

> 4-ounce salmon fillet
> 1 teaspoon extra-virgin olive oil
> Sea salt and ground black pepper

For the Brussels Sprouts

> ½ cup halved Brussels sprouts
> ½ teaspoon extra-virgin olive oil
> Salt and pepper

For the Sweet Potato

> 1 medium sweet potato, peeled and cubed
> Sea salt and ground black pepper

For the Green Beans

> ½ cup trimmed green beans

1. For the salmon: Preheat the oven to 400°F (200°C). Rub the salmon fillet with 1 teaspoon olive oil and season with salt and pepper. Place the salmon on a baking sheet and bake for 12 to 15 minutes or until the salmon flakes easily with a fork.
2. For the Brussels sprouts: Toss the Brussels sprouts with ½ teaspoon olive oil, salt, and pepper. Spread them out on a baking sheet and roast for 20 to 25 minutes, flipping halfway through, until crispy and tender.
3. For the sweet potato: Bring a pot of water to a boil and add the cubed sweet potato. Boil for 12 to 15 minutes or until fork-tender. Drain and mash the sweet potato with a fork or masher. Season with salt and pepper.
4. For the green beans: While the salmon and Brussels sprouts are cooking, steam the green beans for about 4 to 5 minutes or until tender but still vibrant green.
5. Serve the baked salmon alongside the roasted Brussels sprouts, mashed sweet potato, and steamed green beans.

SERVING/STORAGE:
Salmon and sides are best fresh but store well refrigerated for 3 to 4 days.
Reheat gently to avoid drying out the fish or overcooking the veggies.

Grilled Cod with Mashed Cauliflower, Roasted Zucchini, and Steamed Asparagus

A tasty white fish paired with delicious vegetables in this low-calorie combo. Great for when you want something on the lighter side.

Yield: 1 serving | Total Time: 25 minutes
Calories: 185 | Protein: 24g | Fiber: 4g

For the Cod

> 4-ounce cod fillet
> 1 teaspoon extra-virgin olive oil
> Sea salt and ground black pepper

For the Cauliflower

> ½ head cauliflower, cut into florets
> Sea salt and ground black pepper
> Extra-virgin olive oil

For the Zucchini

> 1 medium zucchini, sliced
> 1 teaspoon extra-virgin olive oil
> Sea salt and ground black pepper

For the Asparagus

> ½ cup trimmed asparagus

Fermented vegetables (like kimchi or sauerkraut, optional)

1. For the cod: Preheat your grill or grill pan over medium heat. Rub the cod fillet with olive oil and season with salt and pepper. Grill the cod for 3 to 4 minutes per side until it flakes easily with a fork.
2. For the mashed cauliflower: Steam the cauliflower florets for about 10 minutes until tender. Mash the cauliflower with a fork or potato masher. Season with salt, pepper, and a drizzle of olive oil.

3. For the zucchini: Preheat the oven to 400°F (200°C). Toss the zucchini slices with the olive oil, salt, and pepper. Spread out evenly on a baking sheet and roast for 15 to 20 minutes, flipping halfway, until tender.
4. For the asparagus: Steam the asparagus for about 4 to 5 minutes or until tender but still vibrant green.
5. Serve the grilled cod with mashed cauliflower, roasted zucchini, steamed asparagus, and fermented vegetables (if using).

SERVING/STORAGE:

Cod is best served fresh but can be stored in the fridge for 1 to 2 days.

Mashed cauliflower can be stored for up to 3 days in the fridge.

Roasted zucchini keeps for 3 to 4 days refrigerated.

Steamed asparagus keeps if refrigerated for up to 5 days.

Fermented vegetables keep for 1 to 2 months if refrigerated.

Baked Cod with Roasted Sweet Potatoes, Kale, and Kimchi

You don't want to miss this high-protein dinner option. If you're in a rush, this can all be made on a single sheet pan and tossed in the oven.

Yield: 1 serving | Total Time: 35 minutes
Calories: 525 | Protein: 38g | Fiber: 14g

For the Cod

> 4-ounce cod fillet
> 1 teaspoon extra-virgin olive oil
> Sea salt and ground black pepper
> Paprika

For the Sweet Potatoes

> ½ cup diced sweet potatoes
> Extra-virgin olive oil
> Sea salt and ground black pepper

For the Kale

> Extra-virgin olive oil
> ½ cup chopped kale
>
> ¼ cup kimchi
> Salt, pepper, and paprika, to taste

1. For the cod: Preheat the oven to 375°F (190°C). Season the cod with olive oil, salt, pepper, and paprika, then bake on a baking sheet for 15 to 20 minutes or until fully cooked.
2. For the sweet potatoes: Toss the diced sweet potatoes in olive oil, salt, and pepper. Spread evenly on a baking sheet and roast in the oven for 25 minutes, flipping halfway through, until tender.
3. For the kale: In a small nonstick skillet, heat a small amount of olive oil over medium low heat and sauté the kale for 2 to 3 minutes until wilted.
4. Serve the baked cod with roasted sweet potatoes, sautéed kale, and kimchi on the side.

SERVING/STORAGE:
> Best fresh.
> Store components separately for up to 2 days; reheat cod and potatoes gently.

Grilled Chicken with Roasted Cauliflower, Brown Rice, and Sauerkraut

A heart-healthy dinner with everything you need and nothing you don't.

Yield: 1 serving | Total Time: 30–35 minutes
Calories: 510 | Protein: 40g | Fiber: 10g

For the Chicken

> 4-ounce chicken breast
> 1 teaspoon extra-virgin olive oil
> Sea salt and ground black pepper

For the Cauliflower

½ cup cauliflower florets
Extra-virgin olive oil
Sea salt and ground black pepper
½ cup cooked brown rice

¼ cup sauerkraut

1. For the chicken: Preheat the grill or grill pan over medium-high heat. Season the chicken breast with olive oil, salt, and pepper. Grill for 6 to 7 minutes per side or until fully cooked.
2. For the cauliflower: Preheat the oven to 400°F (200°C). Toss the cauliflower florets in olive oil, salt, and pepper. Spread them evenly on a baking sheet and roast for 20 to 25 minutes, flipping halfway, until tender.
3. Place the grilled chicken with the roasted cauliflower, brown rice, and sauerkraut on the plate.

SERVING/STORAGE:
Store components separately in the fridge for up to 3 days.
Reheat the chicken and cauliflower; serve the sauerkraut cold.

Chickpea Stir-Fry with Broccoli, Snap Peas, and Mushrooms Over Cauliflower Rice, with Edamame

A vegan stir-fry perfect for when you want to order Chinese but also want to keep an eye on your sodium intake.

Yield: 1 serving | Total Time: 20–25 minutes
Calories: 501 | Protein: 32g | Fiber: 24g

1 tablespoon extra-virgin olive oil
½ cup sliced mushrooms
½ cup snap peas
½ cup broccoli florets
1 cup cooked chickpeas
1 cup cauliflower rice
½ cup edamame
Fermented vegetables (kimchi, sauerkraut, etc.)

1. In a large nonstick skillet, heat the olive oil over medium heat and sauté the mushrooms, snap peas, and broccoli for 5 to 7 minutes until tender. Add the chickpeas and cook for an additional 2 to 3 minutes.
2. Cook the cauliflower rice according to package instructions (or sauté in a pan with a bit of olive oil for 3 to 5 minutes).
3. Serve the chickpea stir-fry over the cauliflower rice with a side of edamame and fermented vegetables.

SERVING/STORAGE:

Chickpea stir-fry keeps for 3 to 4 days in the fridge.
Cauliflower rice is best fresh but can be stored for 3 to 4 days.
Edamame and fermented veggies store well for several days
(1 to 2 months for fermented items).

Stuffed Peppers

One of my personal favorite dinners, and it's perfect for meal prepping lunches to take to work as well. These leftovers don't last in my house.

Yield: 4 servings | Total Time: 45 minutes
Calories: 325 (per pepper) | Protein: 15g (per pepper) | Fiber: 10g (per pepper)

1 small onion, diced
1 15-ounce can black beans, drained and rinsed
1 cup cooked quinoa or rice
½ cup diced tomatoes
1 teaspoon ground cumin
1 teaspoon chili powder
4 bell peppers, tops cut off and seeds removed
¼ cup nutritional yeast (optional, for cheesy flavor)
Fresh cilantro for garnish

1. Preheat the oven to 375°F (190°C).
2. In a large nonstick skillet, sauté the onion over medium heat until softened. Add the black beans, cooked quinoa (or rice), diced tomatoes, cumin, and chili powder. Stir to combine and heat through, about 5 minutes.

3. Stuff each bell pepper with the mixture and place in a 3-quart baking dish. Cover with foil and bake for 25 to 30 minutes until the peppers are tender.
4. Add nutritional yeast and cilantro before serving.

SERVING/STORAGE:
Store cooked stuffed peppers in an airtight container in the fridge for up to 4 days.
Reheat in the microwave or oven before serving.
Can be frozen for up to 1 month (wrap individually for best results).

Baked Tempeh with Zucchini Noodles, Garlic, Marinara Sauce, and Steamed Broccoli

This is a great recipe to make if you've never tried tempeh. A low-carb, low-calorie dinner with tons of veggies and nutrient-rich ingredients.

Yield: 1 serving | Total Time: ~30 minutes
Calories: 301 | Protein: 26g | Fiber: 13g

4 ounces tempeh, sliced
1 teaspoon extra-virgin olive oil
1 garlic clove, minced
1 zucchini, spiralized into noodles
½ cup marinara sauce
1 cup chopped broccoli florets

1. Preheat the oven to 375°F (190°C). Place the sliced tempeh on a baking sheet and bake for 20 minutes, flipping halfway, until tender.
2. In a large nonstick skillet, heat the olive oil over medium heat. Add the minced garlic and sauté for 1 minute until tender. Add the noodles and sauté for 2 to 3 minutes until tender but slightly crisp.
3. Add the marinara sauce to the pan with the noodles and cook for another 2 minutes.
4. Steam the broccoli for 4 to 5 minutes or until tender.

5. Serve the baked tempeh with the zucchini noodles, marinara sauce, and steamed broccoli.

SERVING/STORAGE:
  Tempeh and zucchini noodles can be stored in the fridge for up to 3 days.
  Reheat in a pan or microwave before serving.
  Broccoli is best fresh but can be stored for 2 to 3 days refrigerated.

Vegan Curry with Lentils, Spinach, Coconut Milk, Carrots, and Cauliflower Rice Served with Fermented Vegetables

This is my version of a Thai curry, and while I enjoy spicy dishes, you can make it as mild or fiery as you wish.

Yield: 1 serving | Total Time: 25–30 minutes
Calories: 366 | Protein: 19g | Fiber: 18g

  1 teaspoon extra-virgin olive oil
  1 medium carrot, diced
  ½ cup cooked lentils
  1 cup packed spinach
  ½ cup coconut milk
  1 cup cauliflower rice
  1 cup sliced green beans
  Fermented vegetables (see page 193)

1. In a nonstick skillet heat the olive oil over medium heat and sauté the carrots for 3 minutes. Add the cooked lentils, spinach, and coconut milk. Simmer for 5 to 7 minutes until the curry thickens.
2. Cook the cauliflower rice according to package instructions.
3. Serve the curry over the cauliflower rice with a side of steamed green beans and fermented vegetables.

SERVING/STORAGE:
  Curry can be stored in an airtight container for up to 3 days in the fridge.

Cauliflower rice can be stored for 3 to 4 days in the fridge. Fermented veggies can be refrigerated for 1 to 2 months. Reheat gently before serving.

Black Bean and Sweet Potato Stir-Fry with Roasted Zucchini and Garlic Over Cauliflower Rice with Fermented Vegetables

A versatile stir-fry that you can customize with seasonings of your choice. If you're feeling up for it, consider adding taco seasoning for some Southwestern flair!

Yield: 1 serving | Total Time: 30 minutes
Calories: 303 | Protein: 14g | Fiber: 13g

1 teaspoon extra-virgin olive oil
1 garlic clove, minced
1 medium sweet potato, diced
1 zucchini, sliced
½ cup cooked black beans
1 cup cauliflower rice
1 cup sliced green beans
4 asparagus spears
Fermented vegetables (see page 193)

1. In a nonstick skillet heat the olive oil over medium heat. Add the garlic and cook for 1 minute until golden brown. Add the sweet potato and cook for 10 minutes until tender. Add the zucchini and black beans and cook for another 5 minutes until tender.
2. Cook the cauliflower rice according to package instructions.
3. Serve the stir-fry over cauliflower rice with a side of steamed asparagus and fermented vegetables.

SERVING/STORAGE:
Stir-fry and cauliflower rice can be stored in an airtight container for 3 to 4 days in the fridge.
Fermented vegetables can be kept refrigerated for 1 to 2 months.
Reheat the stir-fry before serving for best taste and texture.

Grilled Tempeh with Roasted Brussels Sprouts, Sweet Potato, and Sauerkraut

This simple dish is rich in protein, a perfect meal to wind down your day.

Yield: 1 serving | Total Time: 30–35 minutes
Calories: 530 | Protein: 31g | Fiber: 16g

> 4 ounces tempeh, sliced
> 1 teaspoon extra-virgin olive oil, plus more for tossing
> Salt and pepper
> ½ cup halved Brussels sprouts
> ½ medium sweet potato, cut into wedges
> ¼ cup sauerkraut

1. Preheat your grill or grill pan over medium-high heat. Brush the tempeh with olive oil and season with salt and pepper. Grill for 3 to 4 minutes per side until crispy.
2. Preheat the oven to 400°F (200°C). Toss the Brussels sprouts and sweet potato wedges with olive oil, salt, and pepper. Spread them evenly on a baking sheet and roast for 20 to 25 minutes, flipping halfway through, until desired tenderness.
3. Plate the grilled tempeh with the roasted Brussels sprouts and sweet potato. Serve sauerkraut on the side for probiotics.

SERVING/STORAGE:
> Best enjoyed fresh.
> Tempeh and veggies can be prepped and stored for up to 3 days in refrigerator.
> Reheat before serving; keep sauerkraut cold.

Vegan Chili with Kidney Beans, Black Beans, and Quinoa

I *love* chili, and this vegan version is to die for. Make it as spicy or mild as you desire.

Yield: 1 serving | Total Time: 25–30 minutes
Calories: 530 | Protein: 32g | Fiber:16g

> 1 tablespoon extra-virgin olive oil
> ¼ cup diced onion
> ¼ cup diced bell pepper
> ¼ cup diced tomatoes
> ½ cup cooked kidney beans
> ½ cup canned black beans
> ¼ cup canned corn
> 1 teaspoon chili powder
> 1 teaspoon ground cumin
> ½ cup cooked quinoa
> ¼ cup sauerkraut

1. In a large pot, heat the olive oil over medium heat. Add the onions and peppers and sauté for 2 to 3 minutes. Add the tomatoes, kidney beans, black beans, corn, chili powder, and cumin. Simmer for 15 to 20 minutes, stirring occasionally.
2. Spoon the chili into a bowl and serve with cooked quinoa on the side. Add sauerkraut as a topping or on the side for probiotics.

SERVING/STORAGE:
> Store the chili and quinoa separately for up to 3 days in the fridge.
> Reheat before serving.
> Keep the sauerkraut cold.

Grass-Fed Steak with Roasted Vegetables and Mashed Cauliflower

This hearty steak dinner is high in protein and so yummy your kids won't even complain about having to eat their veggies.

Yield: 1 serving | Total Time: ~30 minutes
Calories: 378 | Protein: 33g | Fiber: 10g

    4 ounces grass-fed steak
    1 cup chopped broccoli florets
    1 cup halved Brussels sprouts
    1 clove garlic, minced
    1 tablespoon extra-virgin olive oil
    Sea salt and ground black pepper
    ½ cup chopped cauliflower florets
    1 tablespoon ground flaxseed

1. In a skillet pan-sear the steak at medium-high heat for 4 to 5 minutes per side for medium-rare (or to your preferred doneness).
2. Preheat the oven to 400°F (200°C). Toss the broccoli, Brussels sprouts, and garlic with olive oil, salt, and pepper. Spread out evenly on a baking sheet and roast for 20 to 25 minutes, flipping halfway, until desired tenderness.
3. Add a tablespoon of water to a saucepan and steam the cauliflower florets on medium heat for about 10 minutes until tender. Mash with a fork or potato masher and stir in the ground flaxseed.
4. Serve the grass-fed steak with the roasted vegetables and mashed cauliflower.

SERVING/STORAGE:
Steak and veggies can be stored for up to 3 days in the fridge. Mashed cauliflower stores well for 2 to 3 days in the fridge. Reheat gently before serving.

Grass-Fed Steak with Roasted Brussels Sprouts, Mashed Rutabaga, and Steamed Green Beans

This is another great steak dinner option that is high in protein and paired with lots of green veggies for added fiber.

Yield: 1 serving | Total Time: 30–35 minutes
Calories: 367 | Protein: 31g | Fiber: 10g

4 ounces grass-fed steak
1 cup halved Brussels sprouts
1 tablespoon extra-virgin olive oil
Sea salt and ground black pepper
1 medium rutabaga, peeled and cubed
½ cup green beans, washed and trimmed

1. In a skillet, pan-sear the steak at medium-high heat for 4 to 5 minutes per side for medium-rare (or to your preferred doneness).
2. Preheat the oven to 400°F (200°C). Toss the Brussels sprouts with olive oil, salt, and pepper. Spread them out on a baking sheet and roast for 20 to 25 minutes until desired tenderness.
3. In a medium saucepan over high heat, boil the rutabaga cubes for 15 to 20 minutes or until tender. Use enough water so all of the rutabaga is covered. Mash with a fork or potato masher. Season with salt and pepper to taste.
4. Add a tablespoon of water to a saucepan and steam the green beans on medium heat for 4 to 5 minutes until tender.
5. Serve the steak with the roasted Brussels sprouts, mashed rutabaga, and steamed green beans.

SERVING/STORAGE:

Steak and vegetables can be stored for up to 3 days in the fridge.
Mashed rutabaga can be made ahead and reheated.
Green beans are best steamed fresh but can be stored and reheated gently.

Grilled Cod with Roasted Brussels Sprouts, Mashed Sweet Potato, and Steamed Broccoli

Perfect as a quick-and-easy sheet-pan dinner or for entertaining guests—you'll want to bookmark this light and nutritious dinner for later.

Yield: 1 serving | Total Time: ~35 minutes
Calories: 256 | Protein: 28g | Fiber: 9g

> 4-ounce cod fillet
> 1 cup halved Brussels sprouts
> 1 teaspoon extra-virgin olive oil
> Sea salt and ground black pepper
> 1 medium sweet potato, peeled and cubed
> 1 cup chopped broccoli florets

1. Preheat the grill or grill pan over medium heat. Grill the cod for about 3 to 4 minutes per side or until it flakes easily with a fork.
2. Preheat the oven to 400°F (200°C). Toss the Brussels sprouts with olive oil, salt, and pepper. Spread them out on a baking sheet and roast for 20 to 25 minutes or until desired tenderness.
3. In a medium saucepan over medium heat, boil the sweet potato cubes for about 15 minutes until tender. Mash with a fork or potato masher and add salt and pepper to taste.
4. Add a tablespoon of water to a saucepan and steam the broccoli for 4 to 5 minutes, covered on medium-high heat, or until bright green and tender.
5. Serve the grilled cod with the roasted Brussels sprouts, mashed sweet potato, and steamed broccoli.

SERVING/STORAGE:
> Fish and veggies can be prepped and stored up to 2 days in fridge.
> Reheat gently to avoid overcooking the cod.
> Sweet potato mash can also be made in batches and frozen.

Grilled Salmon with Roasted Cauliflower, Steamed Asparagus, Fermented Vegetables, and Mashed Sweet Potato

Grilled salmon never sounded so good, and this recipe has enough probiotics to help you reach your 30–30–3 target for the day.

Yield: 1 serving | Total Time: ~35 minutes
Calories: 405 | Protein: 29g | Fiber: 6g

> 4-ounce salmon fillet
> 1 cup chopped cauliflower florets
> 1 teaspoon extra-virgin olive oil
> Sea salt and ground black pepper
> ½ cup trimmed and chopped asparagus
> 1 medium sweet potato, peeled and cubed
> Fermented vegetables (see page 193)

1. Preheat the grill or grill pan over medium heat. Grill the salmon for 3 to 4 minutes per side or until it flakes easily with a fork.
2. Preheat the oven to 400°F (200°C). Toss the cauliflower with olive oil, salt, and pepper. Spread the pieces out on a baking sheet and roast for 20 to 25 minutes until desired tenderness.
3. Add a tablespoon of water to a saucepan and cover the asparagus, steaming for 4 to 5 minutes or until tender.
4. In a medium saucepan over high heat, boil the sweet potato cubes for 15 to 20 minutes until tender. Mash with a fork or potato masher, and add salt and pepper to taste.
5. Serve the grilled salmon with the roasted cauliflower, steamed asparagus, mashed sweet potato, and fermented vegetables.

SERVING/STORAGE:
 Salmon and sides can be stored for up to 4 days in the fridge.
 Fermented vegetables will last for 1 to 2 months in the fridge.

Baked Salmon with Mashed Rutabaga, Roasted Brussels Sprouts, and Steamed Asparagus

A guilt-free decadent salmon dinner. You'll want seconds or maybe thirds!

Yield: 1 serving | Total Time: ~35 minutes
Calories: 367 | Protein: 31g | Fiber: 10g

4-ounce salmon fillet
1 cup halved Brussels sprouts
Extra-virgin olive oil
1 medium rutabaga, peeled and cubed
½ cup trimmed and chopped asparagus

1. Preheat the oven to 400°F (200°C). Place the salmon on a baking sheet and bake for 12 to 15 minutes until it flakes easily with a fork.
2. Toss the Brussels sprouts with olive oil, salt, and pepper. Spread the pieces out on a baking sheet and roast for 20 to 25 minutes at 400°F (200°C).
3. In a medium saucepan over medium-high heat, boil the rutabaga cubes for 15 to 20 minutes, then mash with a fork or potato masher.
4. Add a tablespoon of water to a saucepan and steam asparagus for 4 to 5 minutes covered and on medium-high heat or until tender.
5. Serve the baked salmon with roasted Brussels sprouts, mashed rutabaga, and steamed asparagus.

SERVING/STORAGE:
The salmon and vegetables can be stored in the fridge for 3 to 4 days.
Rutabaga should be eaten within 1 to 2 days for the best texture.

Grilled Salmon with Roasted Brussels Sprouts, Sweet Potato, and Sauerkraut

A super high-protein dinner option that's quick and easy to put together after a busy day.

Yield: 1 serving | Total Time: 30 minutes
Calories: 530 | Protein: 40g | Fiber: 16g

For the Salmon

> 4-ounce salmon fillet
> 1 teaspoon extra-virgin olive oil
> Sea salt and ground pepper

For the Brussels Sprouts and Sweet Potato

> ½ cup halved Brussels sprouts
> ½ medium sweet potato, cut into wedges
> Extra-virgin olive oil
> Sea salt and ground black pepper

> ¼ cup sauerkraut

1. Preheat your grill or grill pan over medium-high heat. Rub the salmon with olive oil and season with salt and pepper. Grill the salmon for 4 to 5 minutes per side until cooked through.
2. Preheat the oven to 400°F (200°C). Toss the Brussels sprouts and sweet potato wedges with olive oil, salt, and pepper. Spread the pieces out on a baking sheet and roast for 20 to 25 minutes, flipping halfway through, until desired tenderness.
3. Plate the grilled salmon with the roasted Brussels sprouts and sweet potato. Serve sauerkraut on the side for probiotics.

SERVING/STORAGE:
> Salmon and veggies can be prepped up to 3 days in advance. Reheat gently.
> Keep sauerkraut cold until serving.

Grilled Chicken with Roasted Vegetables and Sauerkraut

This grain-free dinner is high in protein and is a great source of fiber to close out your day.

Yield: 1 serving | Total Time: 30–35 minutes
Calories: 530 | Protein: 40g | Fiber: 15g

    4-ounce boneless, skinless chicken breast
    1 teaspoon extra-virgin olive oil
    Sea salt and ground black pepper
    ½ cup chopped cauliflower florets
    ½ cup carrots
    Extra-virgin olive oil
    Sea salt and ground black pepper
    ½ cup cooked lentils

    ¼ cup sauerkraut

1. Preheat the grill to medium-high heat. Rub the chicken with olive oil and season with salt and pepper. Grill for 6 to 7 minutes per side until cooked through.
2. Preheat the oven to 400°F (200°C). Toss the cauliflower and carrots with olive oil, salt, and pepper. Spread the pieces out on a baking sheet and roast for 20 to 25 minutes until desired tenderness.
3. Plate the grilled chicken with the roasted vegetables and lentils. Add sauerkraut for probiotics.

SERVING/STORAGE:
    Chicken, veggies, and lentils can be prepped up to 3 days ahead and refrigerated.
    Keep sauerkraut cold until serving.

SNACKS

Greek Yogurt with Mixed Berries and Walnuts

A healthy, high-protein snack you can prep in bulk or make as needed. This one is highly customizable based on what ingredients you have in the pantry.

Yield: 1 serving | Total Time: 5 minutes
Calories: 300 | Protein: 24g | Fiber: 4g

> 1 cup unsweetened Greek yogurt
> ¼ cup mixed berries (e.g., blueberries, raspberries, strawberries, blackberries)
> ¼ cup walnuts

1. Scoop the unsweetened Greek yogurt into a bowl.
2. Top the yogurt with the mixed berries and a handful of walnuts.

SERVING/STORAGE:
> Best served fresh.
> Can be prepped a few hours ahead and stored in the fridge.
> For best texture, add the berries and walnuts just before eating.
> Greek yogurt keeps well in the fridge for 5 to 7 days
> after opening.

Greek Yogurt with Chia Seeds and Raspberries

Another Greek yogurt snack but with added chia seeds for fiber!

Yield: 1 serving | Total Time: 5 minutes
Calories: 173 | Protein: 22g | Fiber: 7g

> 1 cup unsweetened Greek yogurt
> 1 tablespoon chia seeds
> ¼ cup raspberries (or your berry of choice)

1. Scoop the unsweetened Greek yogurt into a small bowl.
2. Top with the chia seeds and raspberries.

Best served fresh.

Can be prepped a few hours in advance and stored in the fridge.

Apple with Almond Butter

Simple as. Why complicate it?

Yield: 1 serving | Total Time: 5 minutes
Calories: 193 | Protein: 4g | Fiber: 6g

1 medium apple
1 tablespoon almond butter

1. Slice the apple into wedges and dip into the almond butter.

SERVING/STORAGE:
Best served fresh.

The apple slices can be prepped ahead and stored with a splash of lemon juice to prevent browning.

Chia Pudding with Raspberries and Walnuts

A yummy snack that's also a great source of fiber—and protein!

Yield: 1 serving | Total Time: 10 minutes
Calories: 211 | Protein: 6g | Fiber: 13g

2 tablespoons chia seeds
½ cup almond milk
¼ cup raspberries
1 tablespoon chopped walnuts

1. In a small bowl, combine the chia seeds and almond milk. Stir well and refrigerate for at least 2 hours or overnight to let the pudding set.
2. Once the chia pudding is set, top with the raspberries and chopped walnuts.

SERVING/STORAGE:
You can keep the chia pudding base refrigerated for up to 5 days. For the best texture, add the toppings when serving.

Cottage Cheese with Chia Seeds and Mixed Berries

Not everyone loves cottage cheese, but if you're like me and love it, this is a great snack to help keep your cravings at bay.

Yield: 1 serving | Total Time: 2 minutes
Calories: 180 | Protein: 15g | Fiber: 6g

½ cup low-fat cottage cheese
1 tablespoon chia seeds
¼ cup mixed berries (e.g., blueberries, raspberries)

1. Scoop the cottage cheese into a small bowl.
2. Sprinkle the chia seeds on top and add the mixed berries.

SERVING/STORAGE:
Enjoy immediately.
You can prep up to 1 day ahead (berries may soften).

Apple with Almond Butter and Pumpkin Seeds

A simple snack that you can take with you anywhere to keep your mind sharp and stomach full.

Yield: 1 serving | Total Time: 3 minutes
Calories: 230 | Protein: 4g | Fiber: 7g

1 medium apple
1 tablespoon almond butter
1 tablespoon pumpkin seeds

1. Cut the apple into wedges.
2. Spread almond butter on the apple slices and sprinkle with pumpkin seeds.

SERVING/STORAGE:
Best served fresh.
The apple slices can be prepped ahead and stored with a splash of lemon juice to prevent browning.

Chia Pudding with Mango and Pumpkin Seeds

A great plant-based snack that's high in protein and fiber—and it's delicious!

Yield: 1 serving | Total Time: 5 minutes prep + chill time
Calories: 228 | Protein: 8g | Fiber: 11g

2 tablespoons chia seeds
½ cup almond milk
¼ cup diced mango
1 tablespoon pumpkin seeds

1. In a small bowl or jar, mix the chia seeds and almond milk. Stir well and refrigerate for at least 2 hours or overnight.
2. Top the chia pudding with the diced mango and pumpkin seeds.

SERVING/STORAGE:
The chia pudding base can be stored for up to 5 days in the fridge.
For the best texture, add the toppings just before serving.

Vegan Kefir Smoothie

A coconut-based beverage perfect for when you want a snack but you're not sure if you're bored or actually hungry.

Yield: 1 serving | Total Time: 5 minutes
Calories: 200 | Protein: 0.5g | Fiber: 2g

½ cup unsweetened vegan kefir (e.g., coconut or almond milk–based kefir)
½ banana
½ cup spinach or kale
1 tablespoon chia seeds or flaxseeds
¼ cup frozen berries (optional)

1. Blend all of the ingredients until smooth.

SERVING/STORAGE:
Best consumed immediately.

Can be stored in the fridge for up to 24 hours (shake or stir before drinking if it has separated).

Apple with Peanut Butter and Vegan Kefir

Elevate your apples with peanut butter and kefir for a midday protein boost.

Yield: 1 serving | Total Time: 5 minutes
Calories: 345 | Protein: 11g | Fiber: 6g

1 medium apple
2 tablespoons peanut butter
½ cup of vegan kefir

1. Slice the apple into wedges. Serve with peanut butter for dipping.
2. Pair with a glass of vegan kefir.

SERVING/STORAGE:
Best served fresh.
Apple slices can be prepped in advance and stored in the fridge for 1 to 2 days (spritz with lemon juice to prevent browning).
Vegan kefir should be kept sealed and refrigerated; use within 7 to 10 days of opening.

Almond Milk Yogurt with Chia Seeds and Berries

Plant-based, quick, and tasty, this is the perfect healthy snack for making sure you're getting your fiber intake for the day.

Yield: 1 serving | Total Time: 5 minutes
Calories: 153 | Protein: 5g | Fiber: 8g

½ cup almond milk yogurt
1 tablespoon chia seeds
¼ cup mixed berries

1. In a bowl, combine the almond milk yogurt and chia seeds. Top with the mixed berries.

Best served immediately.

Can be made in advance and stored in the fridge for up to 1 day.

Berries can be fresh or frozen.

Almonds with Apple

Quick-and-easy, on-the-go healthy snack!

Yield: 1 serving | Total Time: 2 minutes
Calories: 210 | Protein: 6g | Fiber: 6g

1 medium apple, sliced
¼ cup almonds

1. Serve the apple slices with a handful of almonds.

SERVING/STORAGE:
Eat fresh. If packing ahead, toss the apple slices with lemon juice to prevent browning.

Boiled Egg, Almonds, Cottage Cheese, and Raspberries

A grain-free, high-protein snack to keep you going until dinner.

Yield: 1 serving | Total Time: 10 minutes
Calories: 289 | Protein: 19g | Fiber: 6g

1 large egg
1 ounce almonds (about 23)
¼ cup raspberries
2 tablespoons probiotic cottage cheese

1. In a small saucepan, cook the egg by placing it in boiling water for 9 to 10 minutes then allow it to cool. Combine the almonds, raspberries, and cottage cheese and serve with the egg.

SERVING/STORAGE:
Boiled eggs can be prepped in bulk and stored for up to 1 week in the fridge.

The cottage cheese mix is best eaten the same day.

Keep the almonds dry and separate them if storing for later.

Boiled Egg with Probiotic Cottage Cheese and Walnuts

A high-protein, grain-free option for when you need a midday boost.

Yield: 1 serving | Total Time: ~10 minutes
Calories: 295 | Protein: 17g | Fiber: 2g

    1 large egg
    2 tablespoons probiotic cottage cheese
    1 ounce walnuts, chopped

1. In a small saucepan, cook the egg by placing it in boiling water for 9 to 10 minutes then allow it to cool. Combine the cottage cheese with the walnuts and serve with the egg.

SERVING/STORAGE:
    Boiled eggs can be kept in the fridge for up to 1 week.
    Combine the cottage cheese and walnuts just before serving for freshness.

Boiled Egg with Almonds

A high-protein snack that will satisfy your cravings without spoiling your dinner.

Yield: 1 serving | Total Time: ~10 minutes
Calories: 234 | Protein: 12g | Fiber: 4g

    1 large egg
    1 ounce almonds (about 23)

1. In a small saucepan, cook the egg by placing it in boiling water for 9 to 10 minutes then allow it to cool. Serve the egg with the almonds.

SERVING/STORAGE:
    Eggs can be boiled in batches and stored for up to 1 week.
    Great grab-and-go snack option.

Acknowledgments

THE PAST FOUR YEARS (SINCE my last book) have been nothing short of a complete 180 for me. What began after the pandemic as a step into the unknown waters of social media turned into major professional shifts, profound personal reckonings, a deep dive into spirituality, and new beginnings in this world of wellness. I arrive at this page feeling reborn: clearer, calmer, and—perhaps most surprising to my younger self—utterly convinced that we have many gifts inside of us, some of which have yet to be lived out. To my family. Mom and Dad—thank you for reminding me that our family always supports one another. We learn something new each day through the selfless acts done for us. To my brother and his family—thank you for your everlasting support. To my children—you are my greatest teachers and my greatest loves. Thank you for supporting me through everything. I love when you participate and are curious about all the things I'm doing. And to my husband, my partner in the most daring of adventures: thank you for holding space for every version of me—from the stressed-out mom and doctor to the person forging into new territory. You are my rock. I am so grateful and love you so much. To the friends and family who have supported me in this book launch and in life, I am deeply grateful, and I don't take you for granted. I know that life is not worth living without a few good people to live it with. To my professional dream team—Heather Jackson, you are still the lighthouse in the fog of publishing. Sarah Pelz and everyone at HarperCollins—your friendship and faith in me have given me wings. Thank you to my collaborator, Emma Kaster—I am so appreciative of your willingness to capture my story. To my team: Robby, Rachel, Juliana, and special appearances by Mital and Amanda—thank you for listening, supporting, and forging this new path. I'm so lucky to have a dream team.

To my community of readers, patients, and listeners: Your DMs, podcast questions, and conference-hall hugs kept me going. You reminded me that behind every data point is a human heart, and behind every recommendation is a life waiting to unfold. You are my why and I'm truly grateful. May these pages encourage you to risk, to learn, and to believe that you can "save yourself." And that when you do, you will find your gifts.

Warmly,
Amy

Notes

INTRODUCTION: SAY GOOD-BYE TO HORMONE HAVOC

1. Jan L. Shifren and Margery L. S. Gass, "The North American Menopause Society Recommendations for Clinical Care of Midlife Women," *Menopause* 21, no. 10 (2014): 1038–62.
2. "Obesity Prevention," Pan American Health Organization, 2024, https://www.paho.org/en/topics/obesity-prevention.

CHAPTER 1: THE HORMONE CONTINUUM

1. K. H. Shinohara et al., "Effects of Essential Oil Exposure on Salivary Estrogen Concentration in Perimenopausal Women," *Neuro Endocrinology Letters* 37, no. 8 (2017): 567–72.
2. K. B. Lee et al., "Changes in 5-hydroxytryptamine and Cortisol Plasma Levels in Menopausal Women After Inhalation of Clary Sage Oil," *Phytotherapy Research* 28, no. 11 (2014), 1599–1605.
3. M. Uloko et al., "The Clinical Management of Testosterone Replacement Therapy in Postmenopausal Women with Hypoactive Sexual Desire Disorder: A Review," *International Journal of Impotence Research* 34 (2022): 635–41.
4. M. S. Hashim et al., "Premenstrual Syndrome Is Associated with Dietary and Lifestyle Behaviors Among University Students: A Cross-Sectional Study from Sharjah, UAE," *Nutrients* 11, no. 8 (2019): 1939.
5. S. Behrman, C. Crockett, "Severe Mental Illness and the Perimenopause," *BJPsych Bulletin* 48, no. 6 (2024): 364–70, https://doi.org/10.1192/bjb.2023.89.
6. Stephanie S. Faubion et al., "Impact of Menopause Symptoms on Women in the Workplace," *Mayo Clinic Proceedings* 98, no. 6 (2023): 833–45.
7. Ronald H. Gray, "Biological and Social Interactions in the Determination of Late Fertility," *Journal of Biosocial Science* 11, no. 6 (1979): 97–115.
8. M. G. Meyers, L. Vitale, and K. Elenchin, "Perimenopause and the Use of Fertility Tracking: 3 Case Studies," *The Linacre Quarterly* 90, no. 1 (2023): 44–54.
9. N. Santoro et al., "The SWAN Song: Study of Women's Health Across the Nation's Recurring Themes," *Obstetrics and Gynecology Clinics of North America* 38, no. 3 (2011): 417–23.
10. Korin Miller, "The Perimenopause Symptoms and Signs You Need to Know About," *Prevention* (2021). https://www.prevention.com/health/health-conditions/a38571118/perimenopause-symptoms/.
11. Miller, "Perimenopause Symptoms."
12. "Women's Knowledge and Awareness of Perimenopause and Menopause Worldwide," Statista, 2023, https://www.statista.com/statistics/1242168/womens-knowledge-awareness-perimenopause-menopause-worldwide/.

13. "Menopause Market to Reach $24.35 Billion by 2030 | CAGR: 5.37%." Grand View Research, 2023, https://www.grandviewresearch.com/press-release/global-menopause-market.

14. K. C. Schliep et al., "Examining the Co-Occurrence of Endometriosis and Polycystic Ovarian Syndrome," *AJOG Global Reports* 3, no. 3 (2023): 100259.

15. P. Li et al., "Perturbations in Gut Microbiota Composition in Patients with Polycystic Ovary Syndrome: A Systematic Review and Meta-Analysis," *BMC Medicine* 21, no. 1 (2023): 302.

16. Y. Li et al., "Effects of Probiotics, Prebiotics, and Symbiotics on Polycystic Ovary Syndrome: A Systematic Review and Meta-Analysis," *Critical Reviews in Food Science and Nutrition* 63, no. 4 (2023): 522–38.

17. Maya Oppenheimer, "Menopausal women wrongly prescribed antidepressants which make their symptoms worse, warn experts" *The Independent* (2019), https://www.independent.co.uk/news/health/menopause-antidepressants-symptoms-worse-hrt-shortage-a9148951.html.

18. Q. He et al., "Determining the Status of Small Dense Low-Density Lipoprotein Cholesterol Level in Women Undergoing Menopausal Transition," *Frontiers in Endocrinology* 15 (2025): 1500712.

CHAPTER 2: NO ONE TOLD ME THERE WOULD BE DAYS LIKE THIS

1. J. McKee, "Integrative Therapies for Menopause," *Southern Medical Journal* 98, no. 3 (2005): 319–26.

2. K. E. Nakano et al., "Reproductive History and Hot Flashes in Perimenopausal Women," *Journal of Women's Health* 21, no. 4 (2012): 433–39.

3. G. C. Herber-Gast et al., "Fruit, Mediterranean-Style, and High-Fat and -Sugar Diets Are Associated with the Risk of Night Sweats and Hot Flushes in Midlife: Results from a Prospective Cohort Study," *American Journal of Clinical Nutrition* 97, no. 5 (2013): 1092–99.

4. M. D. Hurtado et al., "Weight Gain in Midlife Women," *Current Obesity Reports* 13, no. 2 (2024): 352–63.

5. L. Taylor-Swanson et al., "The Dynamics of Stress and Fatigue Across Menopause: Attractors, Coupling, and Resilience," *Menopause* 25, no. 4 (2018): 380–90.

6. C. B. Lu et al., "Musculoskeletal Pain During the Menopausal Transition: A Systematic Review and Meta-Analysis," *Neural Plasticity* (2020): 8842110.

7. K. Ataei-Almanghadim et al. "The Effect of Oral Capsule of Curcumin and Vitamin E on the Hot Flashes and Anxiety in Postmenopausal Women: A Triple Blind Randomized Controlled Trial," *Complementary Therapies in Medicine* 48 (2020): 102267.

8. M. Akbari et al., "The Effects of Curcumin on Weight Loss Among Patients with Metabolic Syndrome and Related Disorders: A Systematic Review and Meta-Analysis of Randomized Controlled Trials," *Frontiers in Pharmacology* 10 (2019): 649.

9. N. Seddon et al., "Prevalence of Female Pattern Hair Loss in Postmenopausal Women: A Cross-Sectional Study," *Menopause* 29, no. 4 (2022): 415–20.

10. R. W. Wardrop et al., "Oral Discomfort at Menopause," *Oral Surgery, Oral Medicine, and Oral Pathology* 67, no. 5 (1989): 535–40.

11. M. P. Freeman et al., "Omega-3 Fatty Acids for Major Depressive Disorder Associated with the Menopausal Transition: A Preliminary Open Trial," *Menopause* 18, no. 3 (2011): 279–84.

12. N. Musial et al., "Perimenopause and First-Onset Mood Disorders: A Closer Look," *Focus* 19, no. 3 (2021): 330–37.

13. Maureen Salmon, "Menopause and Brain Fog: What's the Link?" Harvard Health Blog (2022): https://www.health.harvard.edu/womens-health/menopause-and-brain-fog-whats-the-link.

14. J. R. Sliwinski et al., "Memory Decline in Peri- and Post-Menopausal Women: The Potential of Mind–Body Medicine to Improve Cognitive Performance," *Integrative Medicine Insights* 9 (2014).

CHAPTER 3: HORMONE THERAPY AND OTHER FAQs

1. A. Cagnacci et al., "The Controversial History of Hormone Replacement Therapy," *Medicina* 55, no. 9 (2019): 602.
2. The Menopause Society, "2024 Annual Meeting of The Menopause Society September 11–14, 2024, Chicago, IL." *Menopause* 31, no. 12 (2024): 1100–69, DOI: 10.1097/GME .0000000000002471.
3. N. C. Støer et al., "Menopausal Hormone Therapy and Breast Cancer Risk: A Population-Based Cohort Study of 1.3 Million Women in Norway," *British Journal of Cancer* 131 (2024): 126–37.
4. "Menopause Topics: Hormone Therapy," The Menopause Society (2025), https://menopause .org/patient-education/menopause-topics/hormone-therapy.

CHAPTER 4: GUT CHECK

1. M. E. Diebel et al., "Estrogen Modulates Intestinal Mucus Physiochemical Properties and Protects Against Oxidant Injury," *Journal of Trauma and Acute Care Surgery* 78, no. 1 (2015): 94–99.
2. M. Looijer-van Langen et al., "Estrogen Receptor-β Signaling Modulates Epithelial Barrier Function," *American Journal of Physiology-Gastrointestinal and Liver Physiology* 300, no. 4 (2011): G621–26.
3. Z. Zhou et al., "Progesterone Decreases Gut Permeability Through Upregulating Occludin Expression in Primary Human Gut Tissues and Caco-2 Cells," *Scientific Reports* 9, no. 1 (2019): 8367.
4. C. Belzer et al., "Microbial Metabolic Networks at the Mucus Layer Lead to Diet-Independent Butyrate and Vitamin B12 Production by Intestinal Symbionts," *mBio* 8, no. 5 (2017): e00770–17.
5. E. An et al., "Stress-Resilience Impacts Psychological Well-Being as Evidenced by Brain–Gut Microbiome Interactions," *Nature Mental Health* 2 (2024): 935–50.
6. K. V. Johnson, "Gut Microbiome Composition and Diversity Are Related to Human Personality Traits," *Human Microbiome Journal* 15 (2020).
7. A. Kumar et al., "Gut Microbiota in Anxiety and Depression: Unveiling the Relationships and Management Options," *Pharmaceuticals* 16, no. 4 (2023): 565.
8. S. Ke et al., "Gut Feelings: Associations of Emotions and Emotion Regulation with the Gut Microbiome in Women," *Psychological Medicine* 53, no. 15 (2023): 7151–60.
9. R. D. Hills et al., "Gut Microbiome: Profound Implications for Diet and Disease," *Nutrients* 11, no. 7 (2019): 1613.
10. D. P. Strachan, "Hay Fever, Hygiene, and Household Size," *British Medical Journal* 299 (1989): 1259.

CHAPTER 5: THE 30–30–3 DIETARY FRAMEWORK

1. Institute of Medicine (US) Committee on Examination of Front-of-Package Nutrition Rating Systems and Symbols, 2010, *Front-of-Package Nutrition Rating Systems and Symbols: Phase I Report*, Washington, DC: National Academies Press (US). Chapter 4, "Overview of Health and Diet in America." https://www.ncbi.nlm.nih.gov/books/NBK209844/.

2. D. Raubenheimer et al., "Protein Leverage: Theoretical Foundations and Ten Points of Clarification," *Obesity* 27, no. 8 (2019): 1225–38.

3. J. Ko et al., "Menopause and the Loss of Skeletal Muscle Mass in Women," *Iranian Journal of Public Health* 50, no. 2 (2021): 413–14.

4. Harvard Health Publishing, "The Hidden Dangers of Protein Powders," Harvard Medical School (2023), https://www.health.harvard.edu/staying-healthy/the-hidden-dangers-of -protein-powders.

5. "Most Americans Are Not Getting Enough Fiber in Our Diets," American Society for Nutrition, June 9, 2021, https://nutrition.org/most-americans-are-not-getting-enough-fiber -in-our-diets/.

6. J. N. Davis et al., "Inverse Relation Between Dietary Fiber Intake and Visceral Adiposity in Overweight Latino Youth," *American Journal of Clinical Nutrition* 90, no. 5 (2009): 1160–66.

7. A. Akbar et al., "High Fiber Diet," StatPearls (2023).

8. Emilie Stolarczyk, Graham M. Lord, and Jane K. Howard, "The Immune Cell Transcription Factor T-bet: A Novel Metabolic Regulator," *Adipocyte* 3, no. 1 (2014): 58–62.

9. N. Zhang et al., "Probiotic Supplements for Relieving Stress in Healthy Participants: A Protocol for Systematic Review and Meta-Analysis of Randomized Controlled Trials," *Medicine* 98, no. 20 (2019): e15416.

10. J. M. Baker et al., "Estrogen-Gut Microbiome Axis: Physiological and Clinical Implications," *Maturitas* 103 (2017): 45–53.

CHAPTER 6: TAKE-CHARGE NUTRIENTS

1. Office of Dietary Supplements, "Magnesium–Health Professional Fact Sheet," National Institutes of Health (2022), https://ods.od.nih.gov/factsheets/Magnesium-HealthProfessional/.

2. D. T. Dibaba et al., "Magnesium Intake and Incidence of Pancreatic Cancer: The VITamins and Lifestyle Study," *British Journal of Cancer* 113, no. 11 (2015): 1615–21.

3. A. Bagheri et al., "Total, Dietary, and Supplemental Magnesium Intakes and Risk of All-Cause, Cardiovascular, and Cancer Mortality: A Systematic Review and Dose-Response Meta-Analysis of Prospective Cohort Studies," *Advances in Nutrition* 12, no. 4 (2021): 1196–1210.

4. D. M. Almeida et al., "Longitudinal Change in Daily Stress Across 20 Years of Adulthood: Results from the National Study of Daily Experiences," *Developmental Psychology* 59, no. 3 (2023): 515–23.

5. J. C. Schutten et al., "Long-Term Magnesium Supplementation Improves Glucocorticoid Metabolism: A Post-Hoc Analysis of an Intervention Trial," *Clinical Endocrinology* 94, no. 2 (2021): 150–57.

6. N. H. Hakim et al., "Vitamin D Levels and Menopause-Related Symptoms in Postmenopausal Women," *Middle East Fertility Society Journal* 27, no. 29 (2022).

7. "Vitamin D: Fact Sheet for Health Professionals," National Institutes of Health (2025), https://ods.od.nih.gov/factsheets/VitaminD-HealthProfessional/.

8. K. Li et al., "The Good, the Bad, and the Ugly of Calcium Supplementation: A Review of Calcium Intake on Human Health," *Clinical Interventions in Aging* 13 (2018): 2443–52.

9. C. A. Derby et al., "Lipid Changes During the Menopause Transition in Relation to Age and Weight: The Study of Women's Health Across the Nation," *American Journal of Epidemiology* 169, no. 11 (2009): 1352–61.

10. B. Z. Wei et al., "The Relationship of Omega-3 Fatty Acids with Dementia and Cognitive Decline: Evidence from Prospective Cohort Studies of Supplementation, Dietary Intake, and Blood Markers," *American Journal of Clinical Nutrition* 117, no. 6 (2023): 1096–1109.

11. M. P. Freeman et al., "Omega-3 Fatty Acids for Major Depressive Disorder Associated with the Menopausal Transition: A Preliminary Open Trial," *Menopause* 18, no. 3 (2011): 279–84.

12. W. S. Harris, "The Omega-3 Index as a Risk Factor for Coronary Heart Disease," *American Journal of Clinical Nutrition* 87, no. 6 (2008): 1997S–2002S.

13. R. Zamora-Ros et al., "High Concentrations of a Urinary Biomarker of Polyphenol Intake Are Associated with Decreased Mortality in Older Adults," *Journal of Nutrition* 143, no. 9 (2013): 1445–50.

14. P. J. Curtis et al., "Chronic and Postprandial Effect of Blueberries on Cognitive Function, Alertness, and Mood in Participants with Metabolic Syndrome—Results from a Six-Month, Double-Blind, Randomized Controlled Trial," *American Journal of Clinical Nutrition* 119, no. 3 (2024): 658–68.

15. N. K. Hollenberg et al., "Flavanols, the Kuna, Cocoa Consumption, and Nitric Oxide," *Journal of the American Society of Hypertension* 3, no. 2 (2009): 105–12.

16. L. Munguia et al., "High Flavonoid Cocoa Supplement Ameliorates Plasma Oxidative Stress and Inflammation Levels While Improving Mobility and Quality of Life in Older Subjects: A Double-Blind Randomized Clinical Trial," *Journals of Gerontology: Series A, Biological Sciences and Medical Sciences* 74, no. 10 (2019): 1620–27.

17. A. Nehlig, "Effects of Coffee/Caffeine on Brain Health and Disease: What Should I Tell My Patients?" *Practical Neurology* 16, no. 2 (2016): 89–95.

18. Y. Kim et al., "Tea Consumption and Risk of All-Cause, Cardiovascular Disease, and Cancer Mortality: A Meta-Analysis of Thirty-Eight Prospective Cohort Data Sets," *Epidemiology and Health* 46 (2024): e2024056.

19. A. Crippa et al., "Coffee Consumption and Mortality from All Causes, Cardiovascular Disease, and Cancer: A Dose-Response Meta-Analysis," *American Journal of Epidemiology* 180, no. 8 (2014): 763–75.

20. Crippa et al., "Coffee Consumption and Mortality," 763–75.

21. E. Martínez Steele et al., "Ultra-Processed Foods and Added Sugars in the US Diet: Evidence from a Nationally Representative Cross-Sectional Study," *BMJ Open* 6, no. 3 (2016): e009892.

22. B. Lennerz and J. K. Lennerz, "Food Addiction, High-Glycemic-Index Carbohydrates, and Obesity," *Clinical Chemistry* 64, no. 1 (2018): 64–71.

23. S. L. Freije et al., "Association Between Consumption of Sugar-Sweetened Beverages and 100% Fruit Juice with Poor Mental Health Among US Adults in 11 US States and the District of Columbia," *Preventing Chronic Disease* 18 (2021): 200574.

24. L. Schnabel et al., "Association Between Ultraprocessed Food Consumption and Risk of Mortality Among Middle-Aged Adults in France," *JAMA Internal Medicine* 179, no. 4 (2019): 490–98.

25. Y. Kawano et al., "Microbiota Imbalance Induced by Dietary Sugar Disrupts Immune-Mediated Protection from Metabolic Syndrome," *Cell* 185, no. 19 (2022): 3501–19.e20.

26. J. Zhao et al., "Association Between Daily Alcohol Intake and Risk of All-Cause Mortality: A Systematic Review and Meta-Analyses," *JAMA Network Open* 6, no. 3 (2023): e236185.

27. R. Daviet et al., "Associations Between Alcohol Consumption and Gray and White Matter Volumes in the UK Biobank," *Nature Communications* 13 (2022): 1175.

CHAPTER 7: SUPPORTIVE MIND-GUT STRATEGIES

1. K. V. Johnson, "Gut Microbiome Composition and Diversity Are Related to Human Personality Traits," *Human Microbiome Journal* 15 (2020): 100069.

2. K. Zhou et al., "Gut Microbiome and Schizophrenia: Insights from Two-Sample Mendelian Randomization," *Schizophrenia* 10, no. 75 (2024).

3. Olivia Rogerson et al., "Effectiveness of Stress Management Interventions to Change Cortisol Levels: A Systematic Review and Meta-Analysis," *Psychoneuroendocrinology* 159 (2024): 106415.
4. Carol Dweck, *Mindset: The New Psychology of Success* (Ballantine, 2006).
5. Mel Robbins, *The Let Them Theory* (Hay House, 2024).
6. S. Aydin et al., "Investigation of the Effect of Social Media Addiction on Adults with Depression," *Healthcare* 9, no. 4 (2021): 450.
7. R. Lok et al., "Perils of the Nighttime: Impact of Behavioral Timing and Preference on Mental Health in 73,888 Community-Dwelling Adults," *Psychiatry Research* 337 (2024).
8. R. P. Smith et al., "Gut Microbiome Diversity Is Associated with Sleep Physiology in Humans," *PLoS One* 14, no. 10 (2019): e0222394.
9. Florence Williams, *The Nature Fix* (W. W. Norton, 2017).
10. Simone Kühn, Anna Mascherek, Elisa Filevich, Nina Lisofsky, Maxi Becker, Oisin Butler, Martyna Lochstet, Johan Mårtensson, Elisabeth Wenger, Ulman Lindenberger, and Jürgen Gallinat, "Spend time outdoors for your brain—an in-depth longitudinal MRI study." *World J Biol Psychiatry.* 2022 Mar;23(3):201-207. doi: 10.1080⁄15622975.2021.1938670. Epub 2021 Jul 7. PMID: 34231438.
11. Katherine Boere, Kelsey Lloyd, Gordon Binsted, Olave E. Krigolson. "Exercising is good for the brain but exercising outside is potentially better." *Sci Rep.* 2023 Jan 20;13(1):1140. doi: 10.1038/s41598-022-26093-2. PMID: 36670116; PMCID: PMC9859790.
12. B. J. Park et al., "The Physiological Effects of Shinrin-Yoku (Taking in the Forest Atmosphere or Forest Bathing): Evidence from Field Experiments in 24 Forests Across Japan," *Environmental Health and Preventive Medicine* 15, no. 1 (2010): 18–26.
13. G. S. S. Tofani et al., "Gut Microbiota Regulates Stress Responsively via the Circadian System," *Cell Metabolism* 37, no. 1 (2025): 138–253.
14. C. A. Michalski et al., "Relationship Between Sense of Community Belonging and Self-Rated Health Across Life Stages," *SSM - Population Health* 12 (2020): 100676.

CHAPTER 8: MOVEMENT AND EXERCISE

1. E. Harris, "Meta-Analysis: Exercise as Effective Therapy for Treating Depression," *JAMA* 331, no. 11 (2024): 908.
2. A. Mahindru et al., "Role of Physical Activity on Mental Health and Well-Being: A Review," *Cureus* 15, no. 1 (2023): e33475.
3. Harvard Health Publishing, "5 Surprising Benefits of Walking." Harvard Medical School (2023), https://www.health.harvard.edu/staying-healthy/5-surprising-benefits-of-walking.
4. Z. Ungvari et al., "The Multifaceted Benefits of Walking for Healthy Aging: From Blue Zones to Molecular Mechanisms," *GeroScience* 45, no. 6 (2023), 3211–39.
5. Gail A. Greendale et al., "Changes in Body Composition and Weight During the Menopause Transition," *JCI Insight* 4, no. 5 (2019): e124865.
6. Y. Zhao et al., "Effects of Aerobics Training on Anxiety, Depression, and Sleep Quality in Perimenopausal Women," *Frontiers in Psychiatry* 13 (2022): 1025682.
7. C. Smith et al., "Strength Training During Perimenopause," *Stanford Lifestyle Medicine* (2023), https://longevity.stanford.edu/lifestyle/2023⁄0711/strength-training-during-perimenopause/.
8. E. J. Halonen et al., "Does Taking a Break Matter—Adaptations in Muscle Strength and Size Between Continuous and Periodic Resistance Training," *Scandinavian Journal of Medicine & Science in Sports* 34, no. 10 (2024), e14739.
9. R. P. Patrick et al., "Sauna Use as a Lifestyle Practice to Extend Lifespan," *Experimental Gerontology* 154, no. 15 (2021): 111509.

10. S. K. Kunutsor et al., "Does the Combination of Finnish Sauna Bathing and Other Lifestyle Factors Confer Additional Health Benefits? A Review of the Evidence," *Mayo Clinic Proceedings* 98, no. 6 (2023), 915–26.
11. Kunutsor, "Does the Combination of Finnish Sauna Bathing and Other Lifestyle Factors," 915–26.
12. M. R. Hamblin, "Mechanisms and Applications of the Anti-Inflammatory Effects of Photobiomodulation," *AIMS Biophysics* 4, no. 3 (2017): 337–61.
13. E. J. Howden et al., "Reversing the Cardiac Effects of Sedentary Aging in Middle Age—A Randomized Controlled Trial: Implications for Heart Failure Prevention," *Circulation* 137, no. 15 (2018): 1549–60.

CHAPTER 9: MOVING THROUGH THE CONTINUUM: POSTMENOPAUSE

1. J. G. Herndon, "The Grandmother Effect: Implications for Studies on Aging and Cognition," *Gerontology* 56, no. 1 (2010): 73–79.
2. Mwenza Blell, "Grandmother Hypothesis, Grandmother Effect, and Residence Patterns," in *The Encyclopedia of Evolutionary Anthropology*.
3. R. Koothirezhi, S. Ranganathan, "Postmenopausal Syndrome," StatPearls (2023), https://www.ncbi.nlm.nih.gov/books/NBK560840/.
4. Z. A. Gilbert et al., "Osteoporosis Prevention and Treatment: The Risk of Comorbid Cardiovascular Events in Postmenopausal Women," *Cureus* 14, no. 4 (2022): e24117.

Index

About the Author

AMY SHAH, MD, is a double-board-certified medical doctor and nutrition expert with training from Cornell, Columbia, and Harvard Universities, and the author of *I'm So Effing Hungry* and *I'm So Effing Tired*. Drawing from her background in internal medicine and allergy and immunology, as well as her own wellness journey, she has dedicated her practice to helping her patients feel better and live healthier through her integrative and holistic approach to health. She appears regularly on national television shows and podcasts and in national magazines. She lives in Arizona with her family.